Your Health Made Simple

If you want to learn more about alternative healing approaches but don't know where to begin, this is the book for you! This easy-to-follow guide presents the basics of a variety of holistic healing methods, including:

- relaxation
- centering
- affirmations
- visualization
- healing with color
- slowing down the aging process
- meditation
- healing herbs
- homeopathy
- hands-on healing
- vitamins and nutrition
- releasing fear and resentment
- weight loss and maintaining your ideal weight

Discover how to create health and well-being for yourself—it's simple with *Healing Alternatives for Beginners*.

About the Author

Kay Henrion is an Advanced Registered Nurse Practitioner with more than twenty-four years of experience in the nursing field. She wrote *Healing Alternatives for Beginners* because she believes that alternative medicine and prevention is the course for optimum health in the new millennium. Kay currently works in a private practice and utilizes a holistic approach to healing. Her clients and students have learned how easy it is to make the changes necessary for a healthier, more fulfilling life.

To Write to the Author

If you wish to contact the author or would like more information about this book, please write to the author in care of Llewellyn Worldwide and we will forward your request. Both the author and publisher appreciate hearing from you and learning of your enjoyment of this book and how it has helped you. Llewellyn Worldwide cannot guarantee that every letter written to the author can be answered, but all will be forwarded. Please write to:

Kay Henrion
% Llewellyn Worldwide
P.O. Box 64383, Dept. K427-8
St. Paul, MN 55164-0383, U.S.A.

Please enclose a self-addressed stamped envelope for reply,
or $1.00 to cover costs. If outside U.S.A., enclose
international postal reply coupon.

HEALING
ALTERNATIVES
for BEGINNERS

Whole Body Approach to
Health and Well-Being

Kay Henrion
Nurse Practitioner

2000
Llewellyn Publications
St. Paul, Minnesota 55164-0383, U.S.A.

First Edition
First Printing, 2000

Book design and editing by Karin Simoneau
Cover design by Lisa Novak

Library of Congress Cataloging-in-Publication Data
Henrion, Kay.
    Healing alternatives for beginners / Kay Henrion.
        p. cm.
    Includes bibliographical references and index.
    ISBN 1-56718-427-8
    1. Self-care, Health. 2. Holistic medicine. 3. Alternative medicine. 4. Health.
    I. Title.
RA776.95 .H464 2000
615.5—dc21   00-036535

Llewellyn Worldwide does not participate in, endorse, or have any authority or responsibility concerning private business transactions between our authors and the public.

All mail addressed to the author is forwarded but the publisher cannot, unless specifically instructed by the author, give out an address or phone number.

Disclaimer: The purpose of this book is to provide educational and historical information for the general public concerning herbal remedies that have been used for many centuries. In offering information, the author and publisher assume no responsibility for self-diagnosis based on these studies or traditional uses of herbs in the past. Although you have a constitutional right to diagnose and prescribe herbal therapies for yourself, it is advised that you consult a health-care practitioner to make the most informed decisions. The publisher takes no position on the beliefs or effectiveness of methods or treatments discussed in this book.

Llewellyn Publications
A Division of Llewellyn Worldwide, Ltd.
P.O. Box 64383, Dept. K427-8
St. Paul, MN 55164-0383, U.S.A.
www.llewellyn.com

Printed in the United States of America

To Gina, who changed my life.

Contents

Acknowledgments

I would like to acknowledge the following people
for their part in the creation of this book:

*My parents, for the love and support they
have given me all my life.*

*Kathy, for providing me with the lessons I
needed for growth.*

*Joyce Smith, for giving me the idea of putting
all my thoughts and teachings into a
book that is easy to understand.*

Ed Brhel, for contributing his life's success story.

*Debra Wolfson, for her unbelievable support
in editing, marketing, and friendship.*

Introduction

I HAVE THE most wonderful story to tell. It is the story of someone who had the courage to challenge a belief system—a belief system that had stood for thirty years and had been reinforced by mountains of media coverage and oceans of popular thought, not to mention a sea of scientific research.

I am sure Rachel is not the only person to ever do this, but she is the only one I know of, so she gets to "open" this book.

Rachel started coming to my classes in early 1992. One of Rachel's challenges in life had been maintaining her ideal weight. She had read several popular books on nutrition and was thoroughly confused. You can imagine the look on her face when I announced to the class, "There is no such thing as good food or bad food. You can eat anything you want and still remain happy, healthy, and your ideal weight. Gaining weight has nothing to do with what you eat."

Introduction

I'm sure it took everything she had not to walk out of the class questioning my sanity—but she didn't. She stayed, she listened, and she believed what she heard.

She learned she did not have to place limitations on her abilities. She started taking responsibility for her health and with that responsibility came power—power over her body and how it responded to the challenges of her life.

With a new perception and attitude, Rachel realized that the food she ate was "good" and nourishing for her body, and what her body did not need passed through. In the course of six months, during which she consumed seven cheesecakes, five pans of peach cobbler, assorted pastries, and ice cream, she lost ten pounds and has remained at her stable, ideal weight. No, she did not increase her exercise level. In fact, it decreased as she became more involved with her job.

This success story is just one of the many described in this book. Perhaps by the time you read the last chapter, you could be one of the amazing tales.

When we make up our minds to take responsibility
for our own lives and well-being, we have taken a giant
step toward total health of mind, body, and spirit.

1

Why This Book?

ONE OF THE first questions people ask me is, "Why did you give up years of traditional medical training and stable employment in an acceptable setting to take up something as controversial as holistic health?"

Even as a child, I was always asking questions like, "Why do people get sick?" or "Why can't we eat everything we want?" I was never content with such answers as, "That's just the way it is," or "That's the accepted way of doing things." After going to a traditional nursing school, spending six years in critical care units, and getting my family nurse practitioner degree, I knew there were things about the system that just weren't working for the patient or health professional. I saw people submit unquestioningly to medications and operations that were unnecessary or debilitating; and I also saw good, caring health professionals get off of the merry-go-round and do other things for a living, such as dog grooming or lawn care.

I could repeat many of the horror stories I witnessed or that were told to me by disgruntled patients, but that would only reinforce a negative situation, which is not the purpose of this book. With every incident, I said to myself, "There has to be a better way. There must be something I can do to make a difference."

I went to nurse practitioner school armed with these concerns and still did not receive all of the answers. Even though the practitioner program is more holistic, it is still based on traditional medicine and did not completely meet my needs, as I found out when I worked independently in a clinic and made house calls.

At this time, a few medical problems of my own cropped up. Endless bladder problems were a source of irritation and pain for me. I also developed a small, painful bundle of nerves in my right wrist and sinus problems were beginning to interfere with my busy schedule. By now, looking at traditional medicine from the patient's point of view, not only did I not like what I saw, but it wasn't working for me either. The medications didn't do much and I was becoming sensitive to everything I ingested. I had adverse reactions to everything from painkillers to antihistamines. My body was trying to tell me in no uncertain terms that these chemicals didn't belong. I decided to listen.

All my life, I have believed that if Plan A did not work, then switch to Plan B; but I didn't have a Plan B. Therefore, it was back to the books. This time, my focus of study was on nutrition, herbs, relaxation, homeopathy, visualization, positive thought, healing, Oriental medicine, and anything else I could get my hands on.

I started using these newfound remedies on myself and noticed results. Alfalfa worked for the sinus problems and I didn't have to worry about side effects from the antihistamine. Herbs, diet, and homeopathy cleared up my twenty-year bladder problem without throwing my immune system out of sync as most antibiotics do. I have learned to love my bladder and picture it as beautiful, healthy, pink tissue always functioning at its peak. The wrist problem responded beautifully to white light visualization and positive thought.

These remedies worked for me; not because they are magic, but because I took responsibility for my own "wellness." Some of the effects took longer than they would have had I popped a pill, but they were without side effects, didn't interfere with any body functions, and were long-lasting. Not only have my physical problems cleared up, but my whole mental attitude is different. I am a much happier person now, with a feeling of accomplishment and self-love that I could never get out of a bottle of pills.

Over the years, I have really learned what the concept of holistic health means. The body is not just an entity unto itself; without the mind and spirit, it is just a shell. Since the body cannot be unhealthy without these two parts coming into play, it also cannot be healed without the integration of the mind and spirit. Picture these three elements as an intertwining spiral, never ending, never beginning, and never apart.

Now, the real reason for *Healing Alternatives for Beginners:* All of my accomplishments and learning took place over years of trials and experiments. I realize the average person does not have the time or resources to do what I have done, and that much of what is written today about health is complicated and time-consuming to read. Since I have always had a reputation for making things simple for my patients and students to understand, the next logical step was to simplify everything I have learned into an easy "guide" book.

This book is just that. The in-depth research that went into this project has been formulated to be easily read and understood by average people interested in improving their health. I do not profess to know everything or have all the answers. In fact, I encourage you to be inquisitive and learn more on your own. This book may not answer all of your questions, but if it activates your curiosity, it will have served its purpose well.

The bibliography contains a list of references and even they are not the last word on the subject of good health. Expand these references with your own, experiment, have fun, and enjoy good health!

2

....

You Are Special

IN MY OPINION, no book on total health would be complete without a section on self-love, self-worthiness, and responsibility for self. I truly believe that most healing on any level—mental, physical, or spiritual—has to do with a worthiness issue on the part of the person being healed.

"Do I love myself enough to be healthy?"

In this chapter I hope to show you how important the concept of self-love is to a healthy mind, body, and spirit. I also hope to demonstrate how one's responsibility for self is essential to the concept of self-love and wellness. This concept is the focal point of *Healing Alternatives for Beginners*. Our wellness revolves around our inner and outer selves and how we perceive them; therefore, a chapter on self-love is a fitting place to begin.

We Are Like Snowflakes

We are all very special people, different from any other person on this planet. Our body chemistries are unique and no one can duplicate how we have lived or how we have perceived our experiences. Everything that has surrounded us since birth has had an impact on our makeup and molded us into the individuals we are today. Think of how unique your life is compared to the life of another. We are all as different as snowflakes and just as beautiful and special.

The Theory of Negativity

Unfortunately, very few people believe how beautiful and special they really are. This, I feel, is due to the negative input from society, which most of us have experienced as we have matured. From the start, negativity is planted in our minds and perpetuated. Some parents punish their children by telling them they are bad, rather than saying, "I love you, but I don't like what you are doing." Telling children they are bad plants a negative seed. Explaining to them that you do not approve of their behavior tells them they need to make a change and are capable of making that change. This is a positive message.

Negative messages are communicated to us throughout life. The media seems to feel that important newsworthy items are those that are negative and sensational. Many events in our daily lives are centered around negative messages: a loan at the bank is secured by threats of foreclosure or repossession rather than a bonus for pay-ing the loan off on time or early; many religious prac-tices tell us we are sinners and never good enough to "grab that brass ring." Then, of course, everyone has their own perception of what is right and wrong or good and bad. With all of these different insights, there are many confused and mixed messages given to us and to our children.

Believe in the Positive

Positive thought is an essential ingredient in the healing process. I have seen people come through the worst med-ical blunders simply because they believed in something or someone in a positive manner. Their belief system cen-tered on the doctor, the nurses, the power of a higher being, or themselves. The point is, they believed very strongly in something or someone.

During my years of critical care nursing, I saw people walk out of the intensive care unit who by all medical rea-soning should not have lived. These people accepted heal-ing on all levels: physical, mental, and spiritual. They had tremendous courage, love of self, and a positive attitude.

The Choice is Yours

Whether we have positive or negative energy in our lives remains in our hands. A negative attitude adds strength to an illness and detracts from the power and healing abili-ties of the individual. Feeling bad about ourselves can shut down every system in our bodies, including the immune system, which is one of the most important. On the other hand, feeling good about ourselves can enhance the immune system, thereby affecting the overall quality of our lives.

Working Together

When the negative energy becomes part of a group energy (for example, a medical problem that gets media coverage), it becomes intensified. Many people do not realize how powerful group energy can be; the energy is strong, whether it is negative or positive, and group thoughts can become forces. When hundreds of thousands of people are thinking the same thought, it becomes a very powerful force under any circumstance.

For example, the media coverage first given to AIDS (Acquired Immune Deficiency Syndrome) was very negative, one-sided, and bordered on hysteria. This became a very powerful force that created a feeling of hopelessness in some of the people who contracted the disease.

Healing circles are an example of positive energy. A healing circle is a group of people gathered together to focus on the healing and well-being of a specific person or group of people. I have participated in a number of these circles that have produced beneficial results for the receiver.

There are other people with an understanding of and belief in the concept of self-love and self-worthiness that is so strong that they have been able to cure themselves of many illnesses. They are a wonderful example to others with any type of disease or medical manifestation of the strong power the mind holds over the body.

You can love yourself back to perfect health.

Why We Manifest Our Illnesses

Over the years, I have observed the ability of people to manifest illnesses that exist on a subconscious level into a physical form. Kids are great at manifesting illnesses when faced with a test they are not prepared for at school. If you are experiencing a pain in your neck, look for whom or what incident would be a "pain in the neck." These physical manifestations are caused by the mind-body connection.

A good example of this is the cardiac patient. Many cardiac patients put up barriers against their world or parts of it. Often, they are workaholics who occlude any personal relationships. This creates a stressful situation in the mind and body balance. The physical manifestations of their bodies become the blocked coronary blood vessels, which can cause angina and tissue damage known as myocardial infarctions or heart attacks.

More Reasons

There are many reasons for manifesting illness in our bodies. What problem remains unresolved? Does this involve someone or something else? If we are asking these questions, it is time to be honest with ourselves. Explore all of the possibilities. One of the first things we need to do is sit down and clear our minds; then we need to isolate the problem and the cause. For instance, if there is a shoulder problem consisting of a limited range of motion and pain, is it because someone has been restrictive with us in an unacceptable way? Also consider the possibility that we may be limiting ourselves or using the illness to hide from something or someone.

A relative of mine related the story of her vaginal infections. At one time, she was going through a series of negative experiences with men in her life. In addition to her relationship problems, she was also experiencing a self-worthiness dilemma. She felt that in order to be accepted and loved, she had to be sexually active. This created a great amount of emotional discomfort for her that eventually manifested itself in a vaginal infection that lasted a year. Her physician treated her with all the conventional medications to no avail.

She battled the infection for a year until she decided to be free of relationships that demanded her sexual performance. At this point, she also started working on her self-worth and within a few weeks after her decision, her vaginal infection cleared up without medication.

Another example is a personal revelation involving me and my struggle with resentments. About a year ago, I began to experience stiffness in my joints. It was getting harder for me to get off the sofa and I had trouble standing upright. I kept thinking that this couldn't be happening to me, that I'm not old and I've always been in great shape. When someone told me that arthritis and stiff joints are merely a manifestation of resentments, I started looking for this possibility in my life. I finally realized that I resented a loved one's actions in a particular situation. I released all the resentments and as a result, I no longer have the stiff joints and am back to bouncing off the sofa in my usual rambunctious way.

More Reasons?

Some people use illness for secondary gains, while others use them to control another person or situation. Many are interested in improving the quality of their lives and need something like an illness to get them started. Whatever the reason, accept it without guilt and proceed with your healing.

Love is the Key

One of the major keys to healing is discovering the reasons why you have manifested your physical challenges. This goes hand-in-hand with emotional and mental healing. I realized that I loved myself enough to give up negative weights, such as resentments. Love of self is so very important. If we could just realize this on a more conscious level, it would make us happier people in every aspect of daily living.

You Are Special

Why?

There are those who go from one healer to another without success. How can this be? This is the time to question why the illness was manifested in the first place and why there is not acceptance of any healing energy.

Accept it

We must love ourselves enough to accept our healing. Acceptance of healing is a large part of self-responsibility and needs to be done on all levels: physical, mental, and spiritual.

Healing is a cooperative and creative process that we must participate in and add energy to. We must accept the healing no matter how it is done—the traditional route of pills and surgery or a natural holistic method.

Who's Responsible?

This brings me to another important life concept: responsibility for the self. One of the Ten Commandments states that we should "love thy neighbor as thyself." The key word here is "thyself." The greatest love of self is the act of taking responsibility for self.

Over the years, we have been lulled into a false sense of security regarding our health. "I don't have to take care of myself, everyone else will do it for me—doctors, nurses, hospitals, and Medicare in my old age."

We never know what the future will hold. Medicare is failing, severe cutbacks are being made in the benefits of

12

both in-patient and outpatient health-care services, and insurance companies are canceling policies on people with chronic diseases and costly illnesses. Soon, Medicare money will be scarce and many people will be very disappointed when faced with outrageous medical bills.

Glad You Asked

Why are we letting others be responsible for our lives and well-being? Are we lazy? Do we have the attitude of not caring until it is too late? Are we too trusting and non-questioning?

Throughout life, we often give responsibility for ourselves to others. We are too willing to put the blame somewhere else so we do not have to look at our behavior or ourselves. "The devil made me do it" does not make any sense and is a poor excuse. When we make up our minds to take responsibility for our own lives and well-being, we have taken a giant step toward total health of mind, body, and spirit.

It's Up to You

If our minds can make us sick, they can just as easily make us well; therefore, we are largely responsible for healing ourselves. No one can really do this for us—not doctors, prescription drugs, thousands of over-the-counter remedies, or any other magical formulas that may come in and out of our lives.

There are many people out there who are trying to control our thoughts and lives. Advertising tells us what food to eat, what clothes to wear, and how to manage other areas of our lives, including our health. The media projects our thoughts, ideas, and conclusions, and doctors have been given the responsibility for our wellness.

For example, we are constantly bombarded with television commercials that tell us, "Trust your doctor, he knows best." Without question, doctors have a great deal of medical knowledge based on today's available data; however, they do not always know what is best for the holistic self.

Make no mistake, some doctors are truly interested in the well-being of their patients. These are the ones who get to know you as an individual and are aware of the many aspects of your life. They will work with you in the holistic healing process (mind, body, and spirit) and are open-minded and ready for new solutions to old problems. More importantly, they will listen to what you have to say and let you be a part of the decision-making process as it relates to your health. These are the doctors who do not wish to take on the responsibility for your health and do not become threatened by your knowledge, but want to help you make informed decisions.

The Driver's Seat

No one should intimidate us about our health. We need to stand up for ourselves. I cannot emphasize enough the importance of questioning your health-care professional. Question everything, especially if you feel uncomfortable with anything being said or done. Have faith in yourself. Physicians who are knowledgeable and competent in their field will not be offended by your inquiries.

We can read, do our research, and listen to all the opinions and perceptions but, in the long run, we need to decide what is best for us and follow through. We have the ultimate ability to create our own lives and realities

Unfortunately, we sometimes get bogged down with the ins and outs of everyday living and do not make our health a high priority. My advice? Quit looking for science to come up with a miracle drug that will cure all illnesses and solve all problems. It doesn't exist now and never will. That miracle drug is *you!*

You have the ability to take charge of your life.

Taking charge of your life is believing in yourself, just as loving yourself is believing in yourself. There are many guidelines to healing. To make the best use of them, you must believe in yourself and your ability to create your own reality. Any doctor who is honest will tell you that he does nothing to actually heal you, but provides the vehicle for your self-confidence, mind, and body to take over.

Steps to Assuming Responsibility

Erase all of the old negative thoughts that limit your natural abilities. We *do* have the ability to heal ourselves. These abilities surface when we eliminate limiting words and thoughts.

Another step for self-responsibility is not buying into another person's problems and realities. For example, I am an avid ice cream lover and can think of nothing better than diving into an ice-cold dish of it on a hot day. The colder, the better. One day, someone told me that I should not eat anything that is cold too fast because it would give me a terrific headache. I had never heard of this before, but I must have believed it. The next time I ate the cold ice cream, sure enough, I got a headache. It took me a while to realize that I didn't need to accept this as truth and I decided the headache was not part of my reality. I immediately stopped having the headaches.

Another example is fluorescent lighting. Same story—I had never felt any difference in my energy level when I was around fluorescent lighting until someone told me it could drain a person's energy. I believed the theory for a couple of years until I finally got tired of it.

Freedom of Choice

There are so many messages in our world with limiting negativity attached to them. I have reached the point of not accepting these kinds of limitations into my life. I wrap myself in white light (the significance of white light is explained in the color chapter) and *feel* protected and surrounded with loving energy and health. I now decide, on a conscious level, what feels comfortable or uncomfortable for me and I eliminate what feels uncomfortable.

When we refuse to accept negativity, we have more room in our lives for positive thoughts and experiences. Getting rid of our fears can free us from many of our limitations. Ask anyone who has ever done a "fire walk" about ridding themselves of fear. These people have released their fear of the burning embers and trotted across the hot coal beds without any injury to their feet.

Remember that the releasing of all negative thoughts must be done on all three levels—the body, mind, and spirit. When we become more open, listen to ourselves, and believe in ourselves, we find that all of our solutions are usually at our fingertips.

The Truth

Perhaps all of the concepts I am presenting cannot be proven scientifically, but they are methods that work for me and other people who use them. It is so important to get in touch with our inner selves and have faith in ourselves and our judgment. What rings true for ourselves is the truth for our lives and world.

The Power of Affirmations

Thoughts and words are very powerful instruments. They are the tools with which we create the world we live in and our reality. What we think and talk about becomes what we focus on, and what we focus on becomes manifest in the three-dimensional reality. Look around—the choice for positive or negative energy remains in our hands.

Affirmations must be stated in the present tense. Begin your affirmations with the words "I am." Be careful not to start your affirmations with "I am going to," or "I am trying" because this puts it out in the future. You may never get around to it. Examples of affirmations are spread throughout the book.

Thoughts Are Things

What we think, we can create. Everything around us was once someone's thought. Everything we see was once someone's dream. In order to create or manifest something in our lives, it must be thought of first. We have the ability to simulate this same process with our health. If we affirm we are healthy and accept good health as part of our reality, we are more likely to remain healthy. Our body form will follow our thought. In our brain, we make all of the chemicals we need for our health and survival. When we truly believe something about our bodies, the brain will produce the chemicals to make it happen. This is one of the basic principles behind self-healing.

Manifest Destiny

Here are two stories I would like to share about people who created cancer in their lives. One story involves a man who went to a leading oncologist for years. There was never anything wrong with him, but he was convinced he had cancer. Eventually, he was tested again and the results came back positive. In his mind he was convinced he had cancer, so his body enforced the thought and the cancer became a reality.

The other story centers on a close associate. For years, my associate insisted she would die of cancer and, eventually, she developed a tumor in her breast that was diagnosed as cancerous. This is another example of thinking a disease into reality.

Both of these people created their own negative scenarios. The original thoughts they had about getting cancer laid the foundation for their future state of health. However, since they had conceived the situations themselves, they could also produce positive outcomes.

Our perception of our health is another factor. If we see our health challenges as our body's way of communicating to us, then we will look at health and illness in an entirely different light. Likewise, if we wish to affirm our illnesses, we can accomplish this very successfully.

One of the most repeated statements I hear today is, "The stress is killing me." This statement carries a lot of power since the stage of the inner mind is being set to literally kill. Our stress-related illnesses have the potential for fatality—high blood pressure can lead to strokes and coronary artery disease can cause heart attacks.

Think of the passive statement, "I feel like I'm catching Aunt Martha's cold." We should instead say, "I only catch good things; I own good health and I am healthy." This statement is a positive affirmation of health. Think back to the comments made by others. How many times has their stage been set for failure or illness?

Old Dog, New Tricks

For some of us, it is difficult to change old behavior and speech patterns. For me, it's constantly thinking about what I say and how I say it. I still catch myself making negative statements, but changing to the positive is part of my growth, and I accept it as such.

The biggest challenge in my personal growth has been accepting total responsibility for myself and knowing that I deserve all of the love and good health the universe has to give. Some of this acceptance has not always been very comfortable for me, but it has made me a freer and happier person.

The following are wonderful affirmations to start altering your thinking patterns and keep them on track:

I know I am solely responsible for myself and my actions.

I am a good person and deserving of my life.

My Heart Speaks

In the following story, I hope to illustrate how the preceding concepts work to create wellness for the body, mind, and spirit.

Before this project was finished, I went through a very traumatic time in my personal life. My whole world, as I knew it, was in upheaval. People I loved and trusted withdrew themselves from my life in a very unloving way. I experienced immense growth and learning during that time and had wonderful friends who stood by and helped me. I experienced new personal growth and *thought* I had released the pain.

What actually happened was that I closed off emotionally from myself and others. After a couple of months, I developed a bad chest cold. Knowing illness is not part of my reality, I searched for the reason I had manifested this particular challenge. My focus kept going to the center of my chest, not my lungs. One day I finally realized it was my heart—the emotional part of me—that needed healing. As soon as I could, I went into a deep meditation, sent myself love, and reopened my heart area.

I began to realize that the past had nothing to do with my love for myself and, no matter what happens, I am a good person and deserving of my love. Upon realizing this, I felt better immediately and, within an hour, the secretions I was coughing up turned from green to clear. One of the most important systems in the body is the immune system, and the thymus gland is representative of

You Are Special

that entire system. It lies in the same area as the heart. Feeling bad about myself was impairing the function of my thymus gland.

For me, this incident further reinforces the value of self-love and the importance of keeping our hearts open and loving. The wonderful loving energy surrounding our heart is powerful enough to stimulate the immune system and keep it working properly. I have a little exercise that helps remind me to love myself. Every day, I look into the mirror, deep into my eyes, and say:

I am happy, I am healthy, and I love you.

22

3

....

The Art of Meditation

ONE OF THE first steps toward learning the art of meditation is finding out how to relax, and I mean *really* relax. You must relax to the point where you are not concerned with the physical aspects of your body. By doing so, your attention will be shifted from the three-dimensional mundane to the higher mental and spiritual facets of yourself.

During my years of critical care nursing, I was able to help some of my patients ease their pain through relaxation and breathing exercises. It took a lot of guidance and positive reinforcement on my part to get each patient through it, but it was worth it.

Learning a New Skill

It is important to learn new skills in a calm, quiet atmosphere where you can effectively focus and concentrate. Noise and interruptions will distract you from learning. Also, a time of crisis is no time to start learning the art of self-healing. The distraction of pain or discomfort is never conducive to learning.

A Good Time

Pick a time that is convenient for you to hold your sessions. If you can, choose the same time and place each day to do the exercise. I am an evening person and find that late in the evening, after the daily chores are done and the rest of the family is settled in, is a good time for me. However, you may be a morning person who is able to take advantage of the quiet, early morning hours. When you have chosen a time, be consistent. This is the beginning of a new self-discipline that will guide and shape your life into a healthier and happier form.

Get into the habit of daily relaxation and meditation. You will soon find that it is helpful in every aspect of your life, bringing a new quality to daily living; whereas meditation in the morning will enhance your entire day, meditating at night will help you get a better night's rest.

A Good Place

Picking the proper place to meditate and relax is also important. I have managed to find a quiet part of the house in every place I have ever lived. Many people use a bed or a comfortable couch. Remember, this is your space, so it is inherently special.

Being consistent with time and space will give you an ongoing feeling of familiarity. As time goes by, it will become easier to incorporate this "alone time" into your life. It will soon become so comfortable and rewarding for you that you will eagerly look forward to each session. First, you need to make it very clear to everyone that you cannot be disturbed when you are meditating. No questions, phone calls, or visitors. This time is yours and others need to respect that and your wishes.

You also need to honor yourself enough to create that special space in time. Meditation will soon become so easy that you will be able to practice your new techniques any time of the night or day, or anywhere.

Music Notes

During your relaxation and meditation time, you may wish to have some quiet music playing in the background. I find that New Age or classical music works well for me and many others. It has been my experience, however, that total quiet is usually better for beginners who are learning to focus and concentrate on relaxation.

May I Have Your Attention?

We have always been told to keep active and not have an idle, wasted moment. Even when we are relaxing, the brain is speeding at a very active pace. We are either reading or filling it with visual sights, like movies or television. Our biggest problem is learning how to turn the stimulus off, or at least slow it down so we are able to focus on one thing for a certain length of time.

After you have mastered the body relaxation technique (mentioned later on in this chapter), it might be beneficial to use candles while learning the art of concentration. Before you actually start the relaxation exercise, please remember that as an adult your brain has had a lot of conditioning to make it active.

In order for this to be a positive exercise, and not one designed to set you up for failure, I suggest that you be very gentle with yourself during your learning process. Your mind will want to wander from your desired focus and this is normal. Very gently bring it back to the focus you were on before you started to wander in thought. Do not admonish or scold yourself. This is a new skill you are learning, just like walking or driving a car. Treat yourself gently and with love. Soon you will find that with constant practice, your mind will stay focused for longer periods of time.

Take a Breather

Breathing is very important in the relaxation process. The following breathing techniques are simple to learn and can be easily combined with any relaxation exercise.

- Take a few deep, relaxing breaths, breathing through your nose. Experience the feeling of love and visualize white light coming into your body. Breathe out through your mouth, feeling the stress and tension flow out of your body with every exhale. Do at least three of these breaths and feel your body relax with each one.

The next breathing exercise is very easy to learn and you can do it anywhere at any time.

- As you take in a breath, count to three, and hold your breath to the count of three. Let the breath out to the count of three and hold your breath again for the count of three. As you relax, you will find your count of three becoming longer in duration. (This is also a great exercise for getting rid of the hiccups!)

The Relaxation Exercise

There are many relaxation exercises being promoted today. The method I present here is one I have used for years. It is simple to learn and, once you know it, easy to slip into. The exercise is so easy and quick, I tend to use it when I find myself in a stressful situation. It helps me to quickly relax my tense muscles and gives me time to focus and regroup my resources.

This technique, coupled with breathing exercises, will be the basis for all of your mental applications. Once you learn to focus and relax the outer body parts, the rest is easy.

- Start to focus your attention on your toes. Feel your toes become very heavy and limp. Keep feeling the heaviness until they are totally relaxed. You may even feel them twitching as the muscles become flaccid and soft.

- Now, move your concentration up to your feet and ankles. Feel the same relaxed feeling in that area.

- Move up your body in increments of body parts. After the feet and ankles, go to your calves and knees.

- Next, move on to your thigh and hip area.

- Now, relax your buttocks and lower abdomen.

- Work up your back, relaxing both sides together until you get to the base of your neck.

- Your next area of relaxation is your mid-abdomen and chest.

- Travel to your fingers and relax them. Work up to your hand and wrist area on both limbs, then concentrate on your lower and upper arm areas separately.

- Relax your shoulders, front and back. Now you have made a complete circuit of your body and limbs.

- Concentrate on your neck muscles carefully as this is one of the first places tension seems to manifest itself. Work up the back of your head, following the curve around to the front.

- Now, relax your brow muscles and those around your eyes. The cheeks are next, followed by the circular muscles around your mouth.

If you are still awake at this point, you will feel a wonderful sense of relaxation. If you find your mind wandering or parts of your body tensing up, take a deep, relaxing breath and gently start over. The more you do this exercise, the more you will find that the actual relaxing of the muscles takes less and less time to accomplish. Also, while you are making your trip up the body, remember to keep the preceding parts relaxed. As your focus and concentration improves, this will not be a problem.

This exercise is important not just for relaxation purposes, but as a foundation for the isolated body control that you will learn later. Keep practicing this exercise until you are able to totally relax your entire body within five seconds. I cannot tell you how long it will take you to attain this feat, as it is a highly individual matter. Some people seem to learn faster than others because they are more motivated by their personal circumstances.

Centering

Before I go on, I think I should better define *centering*. The body is made up of energy centers. These energy centers, called chakras by many, run in a straight line from the top of the head to the base of the spine. A centering or aligning of these chakras usually aligns everything in the body, including the essence that is you, your mind, and your spirit. With this centering, you can become calm and think clearly and rationally. It also serves as a type of grounding with the solid energy of Mother Earth, and involves a focusing of your mental energies. For many purposes, the terms centering and focusing can be used interchangeably.

I will proceed to explain some of the simplest centering exercises. After mastering these techniques, you can experiment as much as you want, knowing that you are bound only by your own self-limiting thoughts. However, with practice, those will soon be replaced with the wonder of unlimited thinking.

Get in Focus

The next exercise has two purposes: The first is to learn control of a singular body part, and the second is to learn focused concentration—a good pain-control technique. One of the biggest keys to pain-control is to break the cycle of constricted blood flow. The more the muscles are tensed, the more constricted the blood flow. The more constricted the blood flow, the less oxygen gets to the tissues and the more painful they become.

Let's start by learning focused concentration on an individual body part. The hand is an easy part to begin with, so pick one of your hands for this exercise. If the hand has a ring on it, all the better.

- Get into your quiet setting and a comfortable position where you are able to have a good view of your hand.

- Concentrate on your hand and every little aspect of it. Look at every inch of skin, line, and wrinkle; observe the fingernails and how they are shaped; notice the color of your skin and nails. If you are wearing a ring, go over every detail of the ring.

- Try to hold your concentration for as long as possible.

- Do this every day, increasing the length of concentration with each meditation. Once you find you are able to hold the concentration for three minutes, start concentrating on the muscles of the hand and relaxing them. Relax them to the point where you no longer feel them.

Hocus Focus

You can use this exercise for pain control in two ways: You can focus on the hand to the point where your entire being is in that hand and you feel nothing in the rest of your body or, if you need the pain control in your hand, you can visualize that the hand is gone—totally numb without any feeling at all.

I know a woman who used this technique when she had a large cut sutured on her arm. It took her a while to convince the doctor that she did not need an anesthetic, but he finally agreed. She felt no pain and recovered much faster than normal. Many times it is the introduction of a foreign chemical into our bodies, such as anesthetics, that retards the natural healing processes.

Practice on other parts of your body. Make this a priority and goal in your life. Get good at it. This is something anyone and everyone can do. If you say, "I can't do it," it is because you have chosen not to take the time and energy necessary to learn. I do not believe in "can'ts," only in "choose nots." Sometimes we are not ready to learn new things in our lives and that is okay, just know that that was your choice at that moment, not that you can't do it.

You can do anything you choose to do.

Negativity and the Solar Plexus

Let me share further information and another exercise. The solar plexus area holds our emotions and a lot of our negativity. Unfortunately, negativity seems to be one of the experiences so many of us deal with on a daily basis in today's busy world.

Either we create stress for ourselves or we are exposed to it from those around us. I have an exercise I use to help get rid of my own negativity. An Asian method designed for weight reduction, I first started using it for this purpose. After about a month, I realized what the exercise was doing to my body and how it could be adapted into something very positive in my life.

- Begin by lying flat on your back so your spine is straight. This is very important because it keeps the energy levels in your body in alignment. Now start with your right hand over your solar plexus area (just above the navel). Rub outward and clockwise in an ever-increasing spiral motion until you are covering most of your trunk area.

- As you are spiraling out, visualize an opening in the area that is getting larger as you rub and a beautiful white light streaming into it. This light comes in and circulates throughout the entire body, engulfing all of your organs, bones, and muscles. It travels down your legs, up into your arms, and onward up into your head. By the time you are at the edge of your spiral, you will see yourself as a total body of bright, shining white light.

• Now you start to spiral back toward the solar plexus area in a counterclockwise direction. While you are making this motion, think of all of the negative things in your life—things such as jealousy, anger, frustration, resentments, self-pity, or intolerance—and concentrate on the negative feelings you wish to eliminate from your life. See your negativity traveling through your intestinal tract, out of your body, and finally flushing down the toilet.

This whole process takes only two to four minutes and I do it before I get out of bed in the morning and before I retire at night. By doing so, I find I have a restful sleep and wake up with more energy and a much better attitude.

Another benefit is that I am also losing weight. I know this has everything to do with my improved self-image. Self-image is one of the issues associated with weight gain because it is how we *see* ourselves. Besides, what better way to hide from the world and others? When we improve our self-image and self-esteem, we no longer do things that add to our size, and can reverse negative actions such as overeating and shying away from exercise.

You can go on all the diets in the world but none will be permanently successful unless you resolve your self-worthiness issues. After all, these issues are the reason you gained weight in the first place. Remember that visualizing yourself thin will also help. Since you create your own reality, you can certainly create yourself thin without commercial dieting methods.

Putting It all Together

When I was fifteen, I was diagnosed as having functional bowel syndrome, otherwise known as spastic colon. It was very painful. This disorder can involve any part of the digestive tract, from the esophagus to the rectal area, and it is usually accompanied by diarrhea or constipation. To give you an analogy, it is like having a charley horse in your stomach.

Functional bowel syndrome is usually a physical manifestation of the stress going on in one's life. The concept is one of taking the problems you are not dealing with on a mental level and shifting them down into the abdomen. For many years, I suffered off and on with this ailment, mostly during stressful periods of my life. The doctors gave me all kinds of medication, including tranquilizers. I soon started having reactions to the drugs and finally came to the conclusion that I was going to have to do something about the illness myself.

I already knew the relaxation technique from childhood (my mother taught me), so I took it one step further and did an isolated relaxation on my lower colon. When I felt the spasms start, I would relax and concentrate on the transverse colon (the part that runs across the lower abdomen) where the pain was located. I would consciously relax that part of my body and visually see the colon untying its knots. I would see the muscles coming out of spasm and relaxing into straight and smooth muscle fiber. I would see the red inflamed areas go back to their natural pink color and the whole colon become healthy and normal. At the same time, I would make a concentrated effort to get myself centered and in control. At first, it took me several minutes to reverse all of the spasms and pain. Eventually, it took only a few seconds to begin the healing and the colon attack would abort itself.

I used three exercises for the above healing: focused concentration on the colon muscles, a relaxation for the colon muscles, and a visualization using my imagination and color for the individual tissues.

Moving On

In learning how to relax, you have taken a major step in healing yourself. By learning the control you have over your own body, this technique will open new worlds for you. I hope this positive opportunity will encourage you to forge ahead and learn many other things that will enrich your life even further.

When we accept the fact that we all share the same space and allow each other just to be, then we have truly evolved into a higher realm of life and understanding.

4

How to Use Meditation

ONE OF THE most frequently asked questions I hear is, "How do I meditate?" First of all, meditation is a highly individual experience. Your meditation time is really anything you want it to be. You can use it for relaxation, learning to focus and concentrate, healing, information gathering, or just plain quiet time. The meditations written below incorporate some of these applications. You can use these guided meditations or others similar to them, or you can listen to music. Sometimes it is wonderful to focus on music. You can also elect to sit in the dark and the quiet and be a molecule. The possibilities are endless. I suggest you use your imagination.

Another commonly asked question is, "What is supposed to happen in meditation?" That is one of the great things about meditation—you never know what is going to happen. You need no expectations; you just go with the flow. When you open yourself up to the energies and knowledge of the universe, you become receptive to all the good and abundance the universe has to offer. It is a time to experiment and enjoy yourself.

There are a few meditations I like to use. You can memorize them, use them in group meditations, or audiotape them and play them as you lay back and relax. If you are going to use them on tape, I recommend two ways of doing it:

1. Tape the meditation as written, then follow it with nice, relaxing music. I like to use a ninety-minute tape on an autoreverse tape player. It doesn't make as much noise as it reverses and ninety minutes is a long relaxing meditation. Although I very rarely use the full tape, at least I know I have it.

2. Tape the meditation as written, then follow it with silence.

If you are using a meditation for healing, a good way to get it into your subconscious is to make a recording and listen to it at least twice a day. It is beneficial to do it yourself, as you will respond more rapidly to your own voice than to the voice of someone else.

Since meditation time can be a time of purpose as well as relaxation, you need to decide what it is you want to accomplish before you go into a deep meditation. This lets your mind know in advance what you want it to do.

Before you start your relaxation, decide if you want to play, do some healing on yourself or someone else, or if you have questions to be answered or problems to be solved. Keep it simple. An overload of questions or problems totally defeats the purpose of meditation. If you are asking questions, remember that many times meditation is like dreaming, so the answers may need to be interpreted afterward.

As you come out of a meditation, it is wise to keep a pad and pencil handy so you can write everything down before you forget. If the answers don't make sense, give it some time and they will. Have patience; remember, this information came out of your mind, so you already know what the answers are. If you should fall asleep, don't worry about it. Your body probably needed the rest anyway. If you asked questions, you will find that within a few days the answers will become apparent. Above all, relax, have faith, and believe in yourself. Below are the meditations.

The Lotus Flower Meditation

See yourself as a beautiful lotus flower, unfolding petal by petal to reveal a glorious golden center. Feel the softness of the petals as they open one by one, each a beautiful creation in itself. Smell the soft fresh fragrance as the night breeze floats past the petals. Feel yourself unfolding and opening, petal by soft petal. Feel a fresh awakening and thrill as each petal opens to the light of a full moon. Feel a new awareness of your senses as light, scent, and softness surround you. You have become that lotus flower. Now see a shaft of brilliant golden light emerging from the center of the flower. It comes up through the center of your being and continues up into the night sky far above the earth. You are able to look back on the peaceful sleeping earth with its green and blue masses covered by soft swirling clouds. Now go into your quiet time and enjoy.

The Meadow with Colors Meditation

This meditation can be done using a variety of colors. I have used blue for love. You can substitute pink for peace, green for healing, yellow for inner awareness and learning, orange for wisdom, or violet for guidance. You may use any color or combinations you choose—whatever works for you.

You are in a beautiful meadow. There is a clear blue sky above you. The grass is green and smells fresh and sweet. The trees around you are emerald green. There is a small flowing stream in the distance. You can hear it running over the rocks. You walk over to the stream and put your hand in the water. It is cool to touch and the wetness feels like silk on your hand. A soft breeze is blowing and you are filled with the feeling of love and peace.

You lie on your back on the soft grass and let a feeling of love swirl around you like a soft whirlwind. It slowly lifts you up off the ground and toward the endless blue sky. The blue of the sky becomes deeper and deeper as you float higher and higher.

You are now in a space that is swirling in ever-changing hues of blue, from the deepest royal to the highest ice-crystal. The swirling vibrations of the blue color support your body and enfold you in a wonderful feeling of love. As you allow your body to be immersed in this feeling, allow your mind to go into the silence and experience what is there for you.

The Living Spiral Meditation

See yourself floating out of your body up toward and through the ceiling into the night sky. Look around you at the top of your home; see the streets and all of the lights as you float higher and higher toward the stars. Now see the earth as a bright shiny ball floating in space. You are floating higher and higher into the endless universe.

Finally, you see a shining crystal in front of you. As it spirals, the crystals move and shine, emitting every color of the rainbow. You are drawn to the spiraling crystal and, as you get closer, the swirling lights and colors become larger and more brilliant than anything you have ever seen. The spiral spins outward, moving constantly. As it moves, the crystals and colors continue to move and change.

You now become part of the spiral with lights and colors constantly swirling around you. You see that the spiral swirls inward as well as outward. It becomes never-ending in its movement, color, and energy, and you are part of that beautiful spiral. As you feel the swirling and see the colors spiraling and changing, you totally relax; you let go of all thoughts and inhibitions, and become one with the spiral.

It is a special place and it is your place. You can do anything you want here: run, jump, play ball, laugh, and have fun. You may also heal here. You can request that questions be answered, or you can go with the flow. Now, go into the silence.

The Healer Meditation

You are walking down a country lane. It is a dirt road. There are tall trees lining each side of the road. It is the end of a beautiful summer day. The sun's rays shed a warm golden glow on the road, the trees, the grass, and everything around you. The sky is alive with shades of blue, pink, orange, and purple, offering the most beautiful sunset you have ever seen.

You are at peace. At peace with yourself and everything around you. A wonderful sense of oneness with the world and universe comes over you. Standing on the road, you feel peace and love wash over you as the setting sun's golden rays bathe your body in a warm light.

You look down the road and see a person who is wearing a deep indigo-blue cloak coming toward you. You can feel the warmth and love emanating from this person as this person gets closer. This is someone very close to you who loves you very much. This person brings not only unconditional love, but a tremendous healing power. This person walks up to you; you look deep into each other's eyes. This person then reaches up to enfold you in the blue cloak and gives you a warm hug.

As you are enfolded in that deep, warm, wonderful blue color, you feel healing energies touch every fiber of your being. Your body, mind, and spirit are cleansed of every negative vibration. You become whole and totally healed of any mental or physical ailment you may have manifested. Now, go into the silence and know that when you return, your healing has taken place and you are whole and complete.

A Beginning

These meditations were conceived in love, with the hope that they may bring you as much peace and healing as they have brought me. They are capable of taking you into a world where you are the one and only creator of your reality. May your creations manifest into your three-dimensional world and be full of love and peace.

5

....

Visualizing to Heal

VISUALIZATION IS, FOR me, the ultimate tool in the healing process. It is during this time that inner strength and knowledge are able to take over and work magic in the body. Since thoughts are things, the body follows the form of our thoughts. The most powerful of these thoughts are the visual ones. It is now a well-known fact that we can cause illness in our bodies. We know that through stress we can bring on such problems as high blood pressure and strokes, heart disease and heart attacks, ulcers, and many other ailments. If we know that we are able to cause these diseases, we also need to know that we can undo them and bring our bodies back to health. There are many tools for health, and visualization is one of them.

Visualization Is Not New

Visualization is not a new concept. There are many books and articles on creative visualization for prosperity, and

45

people have used it for years to reshape and restructure their lives. It has also been used in the traditional medical profession, and there are articles in some of the women's magazines describing the use of visualization for healing.

The Simonton clinics in Texas are using it as part of their protocol in treating cancer, and the M.D. Anderson Hospital in Houston is using the PacMan-visualization approach with children manifesting leukemia. On a television screen, the children watch as the good cells gobble up the harmful cancerous cells.

Even though visualization is a wonderful tool, it is not magic. As with any method of healing you choose to use, you must be motivated and truly believe in yourself and your abilities.

Know you have the power to heal yourself and accept it.

Mind Over Matter

Studies done at the National Institutes of Health in Washington, D.C., and the University of Rochester in New York show that the brain also produces many of the hormones that are produced by the immune system. The studies indicate that these hormones can and do affect each other, forming what is called a brain-immune system interaction. This further illustrates that the brain (mind) does have an effect on the body and how we deal with wellness. As such, we are the only ones who have ultimate control over our mind and our health.

Make Two Aspirin

Let me explain the theory of how visualization works in the body. First, a little background information. The brain is capable of producing all of the necessary chemicals needed for healing our body. Science has proven that our bodies make chemical substances closely related to manmade ones. Some of these internal substances mimic manmade chemicals like Valium and opiates. Two of the most commonly known chemicals produced by the brain are endorphins and enkephalins—substances produced for pain control.

Not all of our body chemicals are produced in the brain, however. Some are stimulated by the brain and actually produced in other parts of the body. One group of these chemicals is known as the vasoconstrictors. This chemical has the ability to cause the blood vessels to narrow or constrict. The amount of constriction depends on the volume and type of chemicals being produced. The act of vessel constriction can be as severe as closing a large vessel to a limb. (This happens sometimes to people who lose limbs in accidents but do not bleed to death.) Or, it can be as mild as a transient rise in blood pressure, which happens many times when we are angry or upset.

These body chemicals are part of the internal safeguard system designed to keep us in balance. However, sometimes things get out of balance and we secrete too little or too much of the beneficial chemicals. One example of this is hypertension, commonly known as high blood pressure. Often, this is due to a sustained narrowing of the blood vessels for a long period of time, resulting in a rise in blood pressure that is not in balance with the body. Studies now confirm that some angina and heart attacks are caused from constriction of the coronary blood vessels rather than blockage. Our brains know when to trigger the production of these chemicals, so it is not magic. It is something you can do and control on a conscious or subconscious level.

The Immune System—Our Hero!

Our immune system is the part of our body that helps us defend ourselves against illnesses caused by outside influences like bacteria and viruses. Basically, the immune system produces the good guys, antibodies, to fight the bad guys, antigens. Antigens are not always the toxins from bacteria and viruses; they can also be found in food, plants, medicines, or any chemical form we may ingest into our body by mouth, nose, or skin.

The reaction of the immune system can be as mild as a runny nose and slight skin rash, or as severe as anaphylactic shock, which can be fatal. The point I am trying to make is that the immune system is extremely powerful. One of the biggest arguments I hear from medical people regarding the concept of disease is, "Diseases are caused by bacteria and viruses." To this I reply, "Why do you want to believe so strongly in germs and not in your own immune system?"

Immunity Granted

The immune system works in many complicated ways. To make it work for you, you need a general idea of what is going on. We have different types of immunities, one of which is our natural immunity. This is an immunity we were born with; one that we choose on a subconscious level to make a part of our being. A good example of natural immunity is people who smoke but are not physically affected by it.

There are some people who smoke for years but have no evidence of lung damage and do not develop lung cancer. Why? Perhaps on some level of their consciousness, they refuse to accept any damage to their lungs. With that refusal, their brain is capable of manufacturing antibodies to protect them from what would be the destructive effects of smoking. If this is true, and I believe it is, we can then consciously trigger our brains to make these protective chemicals.

We also have an acquired immunity. This happens when the body is invaded by a microorganism and it makes antibodies to destroy the invader. The body then remembers what that organism "looked" like and how to successfully fight it. A good example of this is chicken pox—it is very rare to have chicken pox more than once.

"Seeing" Is Believing

There are two wonderful tools for keeping a healthy immune system that have been used successfully by me and others. They are affirmations and visualization. In this section, we will discuss visualization.

Here is a short explanation of the theory of the visualization: When we see an object, we do not "see" that object with our eyes; we "see" with the visual center of our brain. This optic center, or visual cortex, is the receiving end for electrical impulses. The impulses are initiated by the many different types of receptors in the eye and interpreted as pictures in our brain. There are parts of the brain that do not know the difference between seeing an object with the outer eyes and creating that object in the visual center of the brain. The message interpretation lies within the same cells.

If the brain sees a body part healed and intact,
and the belief system of the mind is strong,
the brain may generate the necessary chemicals
and processes needed for that healing.

The important point to remember in the art of visualization is to really visualize; work with pictures. Remember that the powerful part of our mind is objective and functions best when not encumbered by feelings, emotions, or three-dimensional limited thought. Experiments with mental telepathy have shown that the strongest messages received by the brain are visual ones. For a stronger healing connection with your mind, use pictures and keep it simple. As I have said before,

Thoughts are things.

Visual thoughts are the strongest manifestations of all. What you visualize and think is what you can make happen in your life. Everything around us, made or accomplished by man, was originally someone's visualization or dream. If you visualize with an unlimited imagination, yours is a world of unlimited love, happiness, and health. If you visualize with limitations, those are yours also. The day you stop saying and believing, "I can't do that," or "That is impossible," is the day you become truly free

I am even using the visualization process during the writing of this book. I visualize it reaching and helping many people, being successful in its purpose, and being available around the world in many languages. If you are now reading these pages, you will know that my visualization has come to fruition.

Visualization is probably one of the simplest healing methods to learn. It involves little mental energy, some imagination, self-discipline, and initial quiet time to master the basic technique.

A Fowl Experience

To give you some inspiration and encouragement to try visualization, I will relate a short story of my own use of this great healing tool. One night I was broiling chicken in the oven. Using a potholder, I removed the oven thermometer, which indicated a temperature of 500 degrees. I put the thermometer down, not thinking about what I was doing, and turned around and picked it up again with my bare hand. Needless to say, it seared the tips of my fingers.

I immediately applied some ice water to cool the tissues, then I used a focused concentration and visualized a white healing light around my fingers. I visualized the tissue as normal and healthy. Within two hours, the pain was gone and when I got up the next morning, the fingers were totally healed. There was not a trace of blister or red tissue. I use my colors and visualization a lot—they have saved me not only pain and discomfort, but a lot of money on medical bills. Please note, however, that I am an experienced health care professional and feel very confident using this method to heal myself. If you are not experienced, I advise you to seek a skilled healthcare professional for the best possible care.

Many people tell me that I must have some sort of special power or gift to accomplish these feats. The only thing that makes me different is that I believe in myself and my ability to heal, and I quit using the words "I can't."

Stay in Touch

You are the best and most effective healer you know. You are the one who is most in touch with your mind and body. It is you who experiences all of the subjective symptoms dealing with feelings. Falling into this category are feelings like the perception of pain (this is highly individual to each person), fear, anxiety, tension, irritability, nausea, weakness, fatigue, restlessness, and so on.

You can sense when you feel ill or well. These are all very real experiences to the person having them, but cannot be measured on any three-dimensional scale. Only you know the extent of your pain and discomfort. You are the only one who knows when your problem is resolving itself and you are feeling better. Many times, you may even know the cause of your discomfort but do not want to admit it. One of the first questions I ask my patients is, "What is going on in your life?"

Begin to See

Your meditation time is the best place to start working with healing visualization. It will be easier to concentrate and focus on what you want to accomplish. Once you feel comfortable with the concept and begin to believe in yourself, you will find yourself using it quite frequently. Visualization will become a part of your daily routine, and you'll feel as if you have done it all of your life.

Get Tuned In

To use visualization for healing, it is necessary to combine a great imagination with good listening skills. What you are going to "listen" to is your body. If we choose to pay attention, the body will always let us be the first to know what is going on inside of us. Remember that your mind communicates best in pictures and that is how your body will communicate any problems to you. You will need to learn to "see" inside your body, which takes motivation and practice.

Here is an example of what your body may show you in its form of communication: An upset stomach with indigestion could appear as a small campfire burning inside; a broken bone could be seen as a vision of shattered glass; and pneumonia might be represented as a pair of lungs floating in water. We all have cues in our lives that create certain scenes in our minds and it is these very cues that will help you communicate with your inner mind. Maybe your cue for a broken bone is just a vision of a small crack, or you might "see" the actual break in the bone. The more unlimited you become in your thought, the easier it will be for you to tune into the actual event.

Now it is up to you to use your imagination to solve the problem. You can use such visualizations as faucets draining water away from the lungs or using water to douse that campfire in your stomach. Be as creative or as simple as you like. Your mind will get the message and the physical brain will take over to produce whatever is necessary for a physical healing. If, during your visualizing, you remove anything such as a piece of glass or a wood splinter, make sure you mentally dispose of it in a bag or a garbage can; this is a part of releasing the injury and helps to reinforce the healing.

A Pretty Picture

A visualization you may want to practice every day is the one of perfect health. Picture in your mind a healthy body. See it perfect in every way with no illness or malfunctions. Picture health, then experience the feeling of good health. With that visualization and feeling, love your body and everything about it. Do this several times a day. You might even want to add the following affirmation:

I am happy, I um healthy.

Double Vision

One of the easiest forms of visualization is duplication. For example, if you should have a cut on the index finger of your right hand, place the index finger of the left hand next to it. Now you have a healthy intact finger to look at. See the healthy finger and visualize the injured finger looking the same. Every time you think of the injured finger, see it healthy, whole, and completely healed. For an extra boost, you can picture bright white light covering the finger. Soon you will see your minor cuts and scratches healing in record time and the pain will resolve itself almost immediately.

The Bladder of Success

Depending on what is happening to your body, there are different ways to use visualization. For certain challenges, you will need to work on the interconnection of certain organs and glands. A good example is a bladder infection (a good many women will relate to this one).

First and foremost, find a quiet place where you will not be disturbed. Relax and center yourself. You can start your healing process from the top of your body and work down, or proceed in the opposite direction. Either is fine. For this example, let's start at the bottom. This way, you work on the most distracting part of the challenge first.

First, visualize the urethra (the outside opening to the bladder) bathed in a soothing iridescent green lotion. As this lotion covers the tissues, it heals and soothes the burning sensation.

Now, see the lotion spreading over the inside of the bladder walls. Allow yourself to feel a warm healing sensation in the lower part of your body. The next step is to see the tubes connecting the bladder to the kidneys surrounded by white light. This is a cleansing and helps prevent any bacteria or inflammation from traveling into another area.

Shift your attention to the center of your chest. This is the location of the thymus gland. See a large sphere of white light in the center of your chest. Feel the warmth of the light. Whenever you are dealing with infections of any kind, remember to activate the thymus gland with white light. This gland is representative of the immune system and there is much healing power in this area. Return to the bladder area and see the tissue healed with a healthy, pink color. Completely wrap yourself in white light and *know* that your healing has worked. In knowing this, begin to release the whole situation. You may have to repeat this procedure three or four times a day.

During the time you are not actively visualizing, try not to think about the problem. Just release it. You want to give the body all the help you can with its healing. For instance, using fluids to flush out your system is helpful. I have used this procedure on myself with excellent results and a wonderful sense of accomplishment.

The last healing method that I recommend for a bladder problem can also be used as a form of prevention. If you happen to have a chronic bladder problem, use the previous exercise on a routine basis. With chronic bladder infections, there can be a build-up of scar tissue on the inside walls of the bladder. Sometimes, the scar tissue will perpetuate the inflammation episodes. This visualization can help you to eliminate those problems. If you should discuss this matter with your doctor, he might tell you that all of this is impossible and cannot be done. Remember, whatever limitations you decide to accept, you get to keep. If I can do it, so can you.

Sinus Fiction

Another fun example of a visualization is one I use for sinus congestion. First, find your quiet space and become focused. Relax your entire body. Concentrate on relaxing the muscles of your neck, back of the head, and around the face. Now, visualize little water faucets over the two frontal sinuses (located directly over the eyes) and the two maxillary sinuses (those under the eyes). With your imagination, turn these faucets on and see the fluid draining out of them. I have used this visualization several times and receive almost instant relief.

The Spinal Act

I have a friend who gets very theatrical in his visualizations. His style is a little complicated for my taste, but it works well for him. Occasionally, he has a problem with low back pain. He knows that somewhere in the lower back, some of the nerves have become inflamed and possibly even part of the spinal cord has been affected. When this happens, he goes into meditation and visualizes three little men working on his spinal column.

One little man sits up in the brain control room and the others go up and down the spinal cord on little elevators. Anywhere along the line they see the need for repair, they wrap new insulation around the nerves. After the meditation, my friend gets up and is totally free of pain with a full range of motion in his back and legs.

Coming up with long, extravagant scenarios sometimes helps with concentration. Ultimately, you must put a little more effort into your creation. The bottom line is: My friend believes in himself, knows only he can heal himself and, therefore, is successful.

Body Language

There will be times when you have an ache or pain in your body and cannot explain how it materialized. That is the time to really tune into your body and let it talk to you. Maybe that sore leg is the result of a strained ligament. What you might see in your meditation is a bright red spot at the point of injury. When you know the source of the trouble, you can then use your visualization and healing powers to correct it.

There may be times when the original problem completely eludes you. That is the time to see yourself totally encased in white light and affirm that your entire body is healthy. You may also choose to seek the aid of a physician—traditional or homeopathic. Many times their diagnostic skills are invaluable and they can work with you in your healing process.

Lending a Hand

The visualization techniques will also work on others who are receptive and desire healing. I have shared with you many of my experiences in dealing with others. The basic procedure remains the same. As always, you need to be in a quiet place, relaxed, and centered. Enter your meditative state and visualize the person to be healed in your mind. Know that you can "look" into their body. Scan up and down the body. If there are problems, they usually show up in visual pictures that you will be able to interpret. Use your imagination and proceed to "fix" whatever is wrong.

Remember, you are not actually doing the healing, you are giving the other person's brain the key messages it needs to trigger its own healing.

No one, and I repeat, no one, heals us . . .
We are responsible for our own healing.

There are times when you may face resistance to being well. Many people get wonderful secondary gains from being sick and are not ready to give them up. These people need to take an honest look at what they are doing to themselves. Some use illness to avoid facing problems and solving them. Undoubtedly, much more is involved here than just a physical healing.

One of the most important things to remember, whether you are working on yourself or someone else, is to release the healing. Some healing may take longer than others to come about, so you may want to work on that person for a couple of days in a row. You need to accept the original healing and *know* it is working. (Much of this has to do with faith in yourself, which goes back to the concept of love of self). Do the healing and *let it go!* Do not dwell on your problem. Forget about it and go on with your life. The more you think about it, the more power you give it to continue.

Release it and know that the healing has occurred.

The universe and the mind will always take care of the rest of it and us. I have had to learn this lesson the hard way, so take my word for it and make it easy on yourself. Throughout these pages, I give examples of visualization and how I have used it in the art of healing. Know that these exercises are all done with imagination and a creative effort on the part of the healer. The intent to heal and the love that motivates it, whether it be for you or someone else, is a very powerful force. Know that it exists and let it work for you. Enjoy your newfound health!

Sometimes we are not ready to learn new things in our lives and that is okay, just know that was your choice at that moment, not that you "can't" do it.

6

....

The World of Homeopathy

HOMEOPATHY IS A system of remedies and cures now being rediscovered by the American people as an alternative to traditional medicine, also known as allopathic medicine. It is a system of medicine that stimulates the body's own defenses—the immune system. Homeopathy advocates minute applications of remedies that produce the same symptoms as the ailment.

Bacteria and viruses constantly surround us. Many are helpful to our bodies and we could not live without them; however, some can be very destructive if not held in check by our powerful immune system. When the immune system breaks down or gets distracted, even for a short time, we are open to invading pathogens. This is where homeopathy enters the picture to help the immune system get back on track.

Homeopathy works with *us, not on us.*

The basic theory behind homeopathy is simple—using cures for our body in harmony with nature's laws.

Once Upon a Time

The principles of homeopathy can be traced back to ancient times. Hippocrates was a great advocate of this system and there are writings on the subject as old as 1000 B.C. Homeopathy, as we know it today, was founded in the early 1800s by German physician Samuel Christian Friedreich Hahnemann. Hahnemann was repulsed by and became disillusioned with the traditional medical practices of his time. Back then, physicians believed they could "expel" illness and disease from a patient by burning, blistering, bleeding, and inducing vomiting and diarrhea. (If you look at the side effects of some of today's drugs, you may wonder how far we have progressed.)

Getting a prescription for medicine was not necessarily a good idea back then either, considering there could be as many as fifty drugs mixed into one prescription. Talk about mass confusion in the body!

In place of a medical practice, Hahnemann turned to translating old medical manuscripts. It was in one of these old manuscripts that he made an important discovery. He read about cinchona bark, or quinine, which had been used in the Orient for hundreds of years to cure intermittent fever or malaria. The writing proposed it was the astringent quality of the bark that cured the fever. Hahnemann knew of other substances with much stronger astringent qualities, but they did not cure malaria. His curiosity got the better of him and he set out to find how this natural remedy worked so well. He decided to use it on himself. Hahnemann found that in a healthy person, quinine produced malaria-type symptoms that wore off after a couple of hours. With this information and after testing other substances, he established the Law of Similars.

Repeats

The Law of Similars states that a remedy can cure a disease if the remedy can duplicate in a healthy person the same symptoms of the disease. The first known writings on this law appear in tenth-century B.C. Hindu manuscripts. Hippocrates later described it in 400 B.C.: "Through the like, disease is produced, and through the application of the like, it is cured."

Prove It

Even though the concept is very old, Hahnemann was the first person to test this principle and establish it as a foundation for a practice of medicine. The testing was called the Law of Proving. He accomplished this testing by applying many preparations on himself and anyone he could get to volunteer (mostly his family). He tested healthy people rather than sick people. He did not test laboratory animals who could not tell him how they felt or the nature of their subjective symptoms. The results were carefully recorded and put together into a "characteristic remedy picture."

At the time of his death in 1843, Hahnemann had tested and proved ninety-one substances. By the end of the century, there were more than 600 remedies in the homeopathic pharmacopoeia. In the 1940s, the American Institute of Homeopathy started reproving remedies. In doing so, they discovered the same results as Hahnemann. Thus, his reference books may be old, but still reliable and very valuable.

In the United States

Homeopathy was first introduced in the United States in the 1830s, mainly due to its success in treating cholera patients in Europe during the epidemic. At the time, most allopathic physicians in the United States were using large doses of mercury and the widely accepted practice of bleeding to treat cholera patients, but neither of these methods were conducive to their continued health. Homeopathic physicians, however, were using "little sugar pills" to successfully restore health, which was welcomed by many patients. Some of the remedies used by homeopaths were even adopted by allopaths due to their success and acceptance.

As many people chose homeopathy over the primitive allopathic methods, the medical community became ailing in its most vulnerable spot—the pocketbook.

Homeopaths were licensed medical doctors, not quacks with minimal education, and they eventually became a real threat. The AMA was formed about two years after the American Institute of Homeopathy opened its doors. The organization ostracized and expelled any member who would associate with a homeopath.

The Decline of Homeopathy

There were three basic reasons for the decline of the homeopath. One was the change in lifestyle of the average American; it changed to a faster pace at home and work. This fast pace set precedents and made way for the concept of "cattle car medicine" to replace the long, lengthy visit with the family physician that was needed to get a good detailed history and physical.

The second reason was the rise of the drug industry after the Civil War. It became easy to mass produce and dispense drugs in a short period of time. The guidelines were simple when treating only the symptoms and not the whole person!

The third reason was the lack of funding for the homeopathic schools. The AMA, which does scholastic evaluations for medical schools, gave the homeopathic schools low evaluations. This excluded them from important grant money to keep them in operation.

However, despite the controversy and the decline, homeopathy is still very popular in the rest of the civilized world. The royal family in England has used homeopaths for years. The rest of Europe and Russia is very heavily populated by homeopathic practitioners, and India is one of the biggest users of homeopathy.

The Practice of Homeopathy

Let us now take a closer look at this science and the people who practice it. The homeopathic practitioner is interested in the complete person on a physical, mental, and emotional level. All levels must be in harmony for the person to be healed. Homeopaths feel that healing progresses from the inside out; from the mental and emotional to the vital organs and outer covering of the body. If the physical condition improves but the mental condition worsens, the patient is thought to be getting worse. Since the body is viewed as a complete whole, it is thought that no isolated part of the body can be sick alone—all parts must interact.

Healing Symptoms

Take a moment and think back on your own physical problems. Is there a part of your body that the flu does not seem to touch? Now think about how you feel emotionally when sick or injured. Even a simple injury brings about some sort of emotional response. Now think how your emotional problems have affected the physical part of you—tension headaches, stomach upsets, or hives, to name a few. This should demonstrate why it is so important to consider all symptoms. To treat only the most superficial symptoms, such as a tension headache or an upset stomach, does not get to the cause of the problem and sometimes inhibits the body's natural healing process.

Symptoms are a guide to the most effective treatment to stimulate the body's defenses. Homeopathy deals with the concept that symptoms are the body's attempt to heal itself and remedies help stimulate the immune system to do so. Not only do homeopaths look at diseases caused by bacteria and viruses, they also look at the immune system of the person. Since remedies are geared to work on the immune system, people treated with homeopathic remedies usually recover faster than others and are more resistant to other infections.

Antibiotics

Several medical researchers have noted that antibiotic therapy will not work in many cases unless the body can draw on its own immune system. Some antibiotics depress the immune system and some lower the body's defenses against other invaders by killing the beneficial bacteria that normally live on the skin and in the digestive tract. Some antibiotics may cause continuous diarrhea, and the patient may need other medication to control that. These medications are not cheap.

I once knew a patient who was being treated for antibiotic-induced diarrhea and he almost fainted when he went to pay his drug bill. There are also many antibiotic-resistant organisms; viruses are one example. The rare antiviral medications on the market today are not only expensive, but they need to be taken before the virus takes hold. Many strains of bacteria have also become resistant to traditional antibiotics that have been used for years to overcome them. For instance, there are strains of venereal disease that are now penicillin resistant.

Prescriptions for Whole Individuals

Now we come to remedies. For proper selection of a remedy, all symptoms must be studied objectively and subjectively, and the mental, emotional, and physical signs must be considered together. You need to look at all aspects of the problem. What makes it worse? What makes it better? What is the person's emotional state? What may have preceded the problem? What is the persons personality like? How does the person react to physical or mental problems? You can see that all of this would take much longer than five minutes with the doctor.

People using homeopathic skills and prescribing techniques, whether for themselves or for another, must view that individual as a whole and unique being with a pattern of symptoms. Then a remedy must be found to re-establish the health of the entire individual as a whole. The reactions to homeopathic remedies may not be the same as to allopathic drugs. There may be several types of reactions to the remedies, such as:

- For a chronic problem, the initial reaction may be a slight physical worsening but a better mental state, then an improvement of the physical state.

- In an acute case, there is usually a slower but long-lasting relief of all symptoms.

- Sometimes the patient will get better and then relapse slightly. This calls for a repeat of the initial dose.

- Sometimes symptoms change after the initial dose. Here, you would need to reassess the situation and change the remedy. Some symptoms change quickly, as in a respiratory problem, and some change slowly, as in an infection or a cut.

- If the patient fails to respond mentally or physically, it is time to regroup, try again, and possibly seek the help of a homeopathic physician.

Remedy the Situation

I would like to tell you a little about remedies and how they are so different from those of allopathic medicine. There is a common misconception that is constantly reinforced by our society that if a little bit of something is good, then a lot is better. This is not really true of most things, especially homeopathic remedies. The smaller the remedy, the more potent it is. There is no maximum strength aspirin in this realm. Since remedies are a catalyst to the body's own healing system, you would only want to use small doses.

Preparations are obtained from natural sources: animals, minerals, and vegetables. They are prepared in such a way that they are nontoxic, do not cause side effects, and do not interfere with normal body functions. They are also much cheaper than prescription drugs.

In more than 150 years of homeopathic medicine, there has never been a recall by the FDA. But, as with everything in this world, the remedies must be treated with respect. It is important to remember that even these gentle, safe substances can be abused and become harmful. Let's face it—you can even overdose and get extremely sick on chocolate chip cookies!

We have talked about the fact that remedies are given in small amounts and you are probably wondering how this is done and how it works. For one thing, no one really knows how the homeopathic remedies work, but no one knows how aspirin works either. The simple fact is they do work, even if modern science has not been able to untangle the mystery of the *spirit-mind-body-chemical connection*.

Potentization: Quality Not Quantity

This brings us to the Law of Potentization. Potentization is the process of diluting and shaking or grinding the original plant, animal, or mineral preparation down to the point where the resulting medication contains no molecules of the original substance. The shaking or grinding is what releases the inherent energy of the substance. These small doses are called potencies. The more dilute a substance, the more potent it becomes.

The power of the remedy is its "quality," not its "quantity." A good example is arsenic. Arsenic in its natural state is toxic to the system, but after it is potentized it is safe and effective for many cures. Other examples include using belladonna (a remedy prepared from the deadly nightshade plant) instead of penicillin for strep throat, or using a gentle gelsemium for a tension headache instead of as a tranquilizer. A substance can be diluted anywhere from three to 100,000 times. The more it is diluted, the stronger it becomes. Most of the books on "home prescribing" deal with the lower-potency remedies. These work well on most minor problems that may arise in a normal lifetime. Just a small note of important interest about the remedies: Do not mix allopathic medicine like aspirin or acetaminophen with the homeopathics. Also, coffee and camphor tend to negate the remedy effects.

Is Homeopathy for You?

There are many good books on homeopathy listed in the bibliography. I use these books myself for my own remedy knowledge. (I turned to homeopathy as a health alternative when my body would no longer tolerate allopathic chemicals.) I highly recommend them to anyone looking for a safe, practical alternative to the chemicals on the market today. They offer good commonsense knowledge on homeopathy for use in the home.

These books also offer good guidelines as to when it is best to seek a homeopathic physician. If you are treating yourself or anyone else homeopathically, use the guidelines in the prescribing books and follow them carefully. They are time-proven techniques.

The most important aspect in using homeopathic remedies is that it encourages responsibility for your own health and gives you much more control over what is happening to your body. It also gives you easy-to-follow guidelines for becoming more in touch with your body. When you use the symptom and prescribing guides in the handbooks, you realize things about your body you never thought of before. At first, the prescribing may seem complicated; however, once you become in tune with your body, everything will fall into place. There may even be times when just knowing what is going on inside of you may change things and allow healing to take place. In many instances, knowing is the first step to resolving.

7

....

Healing Hues of Color

LIVING ON EARTH, we are constantly surrounded by certain vibratory forces. Our hearing and vision perceive forces such as sound and color, and love and hate are perceived as feelings and can be a strong intangible influence in our lives. We know that certain sounds and colors create different feelings. When we begin to get in touch with the deeper part of ourselves, we realize that sounds and colors can be used as powerful creative forces.

Vibratory color sensation is the highest form of color. Every color vibrates at a different level. It is easy to test this yourself if you are not already aware of the effect colors have on you. Take a bright red object and look at it for a few minutes. Hold it close and feel its warm energy vibration. It may even make you feel more energetic. Now take a pink object, hold it close to you, and look at it. You will probably feel peaceful and serene. These colors are within the same spectrum and differ by only a few shades, but have totally different vibratory energies.

Rainbows Around Us

The entire spectrum of the rainbow is at our fingertips. Not only do we have many three-dimensional flat colors, but we also have developed a variety of light colors. Whatever medium we deal with, color affects us all. Even people who are not sighted are affected by color, if they choose to be. There are color sensations for those who choose to tune into the vibrations that surround them.

Color can express every sensory feeling and emotion known to man. The warm colors of red, orange, and yellow have been used to represent heat, anger, energy, intense feelings, light, enlightenment, and inner awareness. Then there are the cool colors: blue and green. They signify calmness, serenity, sadness, health, tranquillity, water, nature, and coolness. The earthy hues of brown and tan can give one a feeling of being grounded or close to Mother Earth. Many times these colors transmit a homey "back to nature" feeling. Even colors within the same family can stimulate different feelings, depending on their color value. Deep purple can be very vibrant, transmitting emotion and power, while cool lavender can be very soothing. Deep colors, such as royal blue and emerald green, give one a feeling of luxury, richness, and depth. Pastel hues emit a light airy feeling of spring and summer.

Of course, there are some colors that have special meanings to us as individuals. Maybe as a child your favorite stuffed toy was a pastel yellow. As a result, today that color brings a feeling of peace, warmth, and love.

Color Your World

Being the creative creatures that we are, we as humans have chosen to create many colors not found in nature; we surround ourselves with color at home, in our clothes, at places of work and play, in our vehicles, and even in food. Color symbolizes life and energy.

Colors are used to affect moods, emotions, and reactions to situations. Many hospitals have entirely redecorated their interiors by changing the colors of their walls to the more peaceful and serene greens and blues. These are calming, cool colors that have a sedating effect on people who are in a stressful environment, such as a hospital.

Color is very important socially. For example, our entertainment revolves around color. Color television outclasses the lowly black-and-white model used years ago. Restaurants are either bright and cheerful, or quietly subtle with muted colors. Some of our happiest social events are based on color; parades, especially the Tournament of Roses on New Year's Day, base their success on color. Colors can be used to capture your attention, as in advertising.

People perceive colors in many different ways. What is enjoyable for me to see may not be for you. Some of us are drawn to bright vivid colors, while others like muted or shaded hues. Colors also have many varied effects on people.

Without question, food advertisements are among the most spectacular in color. Who could deny a deep, juicy brown hamburger on a lightly tanned bun with a bright-red tomato slice and a cool, lime-green lettuce leaf? The image makes me hungry and I don't even eat red meat! Food garnishes and decorations have been used for hundreds of years to stimulate the appetite and possibly hide the less favorable characteristics of the food, such as the taste.

Back to the brightly colored picture of the hamburger, as seen in advertisements. I, for one, have never seen that same image of a hamburger when it comes flying across the fast food counter securely wrapped and smashed in its foil wrapper. Unfortunately, by then, that colorful picture of that promised "hamburger in the sky" has done its work on you. The vision of a succulent hamburger has activated the digestive juices and you are probably hungry enough to eat anything—no matter what color it is.

Experience Color

Only we can feel and control the vibration of color in ourselves. We can direct the color to do whatever we want, like intensifying reds to bring in more energy (a better alternative than caffeine). We can calm and reassure ourselves with soft pink, and we can love and bring health to ourselves with an emerald green light.

Another way to experience color is through meditation. You can create a specific color, or you can relax and explore what comes. However you choose to do it, it will be an experience you will never forget. To see a color in deep meditation is to fully experience that color. You have the ability to become close to that color and become part of its vibratory force. By doing so, the color becomes almost liquid and totally engulfs you until you and the color are one. This is a totally sensational and breathtaking experience.

Healing Colors and How They Work

You are probably wondering where color fits in and why I am so enthusiastic about it. Color has tremendous healing properties and potentials. These potentials exist on three levels: the mind, body, and spirit.

Color healing is very old, dating back to the ancient Egyptians. This technique is enjoying a revival today by those looking for alternative ways to health. Color healing is not only being used by lay people—many professionals in the mental health field are also using color in their therapy sessions.

The Colors!

What I will give you now are guidelines on colors and how to use them. Although these guidelines have worked for me, you may be more comfortable with other colors for certain effects. For example, you may find that a phosphorescent green gives you energy or a pastel lime green promotes peace and serenity. Whatever feels comfortable for you is what will work best. As I have said before, tune into your own body and inner self to do whatever is in your highest good.

Red: A high-energy color. Red can be used to speed up sluggish body systems or give them that extra boost of energy. On mornings when I wake up and still feel tired, I visualize myself wrapped in red swirling light and feel energized in only a few minutes.

Green: A rebuilding energy. Green is used to rebuild or replace damaged cells. Visualizing green is great for cuts or damaged bones, muscles, tendons, or ligaments. Green can also be used as a multipurpose healing color when seen as an emerald-green light.

Blue: A calming energy. The effects of blue can reduce pain and discomfort. It works mainly on the nervous system. While waiting for your healing to work, mentally wrap yourself or your injured part in blue light. This helps disperse the pain and discomfort. For some reason, red fire ants in Florida seem to find my feet appetizing morsels. A baking soda paste helps neutralize the acid of the bite, but there are times when that is not an option, in which case I use an intense ice-blue light on the affected area and, within two to three minutes, the stinging and burning is usually gone for good.

Pink: Also a calming energy. Using pink, you are able to create a sense of peace and well-being. I use pink for many things; it is great for reducing stress when caught in traffic jams or any other uncontrollable situation that would normally send your stress level sky-high. I also use pink light in treating other people. When I was working in pediatrics, I would wrap a screaming child and myself in pink light so the child would calm down enough to be examined. Doing this has a twofold purpose; one, you are able to remain calm and not feed any more emotion into the situation and, two, the calming vibrations will actually be picked up by the child, which will help to calm the child's emotional level.

White: This crystal energy is the highest of all. When you hold a focused concentration on a swirling white-crystal light, you are capable of doing just about anything. I have used this white-crystal light on others and myself with the most amazing results. I use it for the simple things, such as changing negative behavior. When I am approached by people in nasty negative moods—for example, a clerk in a grocery store who is having a bad day—I mentally wrap this person in white-crystal light and think, "I love you. Know that you are loved." If you feel this from your heart, you will not only see that person change before your eyes, but you will feel a wonderful emotional high that can never be equaled by any drug or chemical.

White light is also used for protection. First, know that white light comes from the unlimited love of the universe. Wrap yourself in it and know you are protected. I use white light when I travel or walk through dark parking lots at night, and I've used it when I'm around people whom I feel could harm me. I have always been met with positive results.

Healing in Color

I would like to give you an example of a healing meditation using colors: A friend's seven-year-old daughter has many respiratory-type allergies. Once when I was visiting, I heard the child coughing most of the night. I asked her mother if I could try a healing meditation the next evening. We did the relaxation exercise first and, once she was relaxed, I visually took her into an emerald-green forest.

In the forest, we visualized a crystal cave. I took her into the cave and had her lie on a healing table. I then told her to visualize green light coming down from the crystals on the ceiling. She was to see the light enter through her nose, swirl around inside her head, and pass through her nasal passages. Then, she was to take the light down her windpipe into the chest area. At this point, she let the light swirl around her chest area, touching her lungs and thymus gland. I told her that her breathing passages were now clear and she did not need to cough anymore. Having completed the session, I left her sleeping. She did not cough at all that night or the next morning.

The facilitator and the receiver must accept this method of healing, as with any healing technique you would do on yourself or anyone else. If you really want to get well, it will happen, and colors are wonderful tools to help this process. The scenarios and examples I have given you are just the tip of the iceberg. Try these and others on yourself and others in times of need.

8

....

Conquering Stress

STRESS. THERE IS so much written about stress today that it can become stressful just finding a good book or technique to help alleviate it.

Stress, as explained by many experts, is the everyday wear and tear on the body and all of its functioning parts. Many talk about positive and negative stress and how it affects the body. There are even lists of illnesses commonly associated with stress; the following are some examples:

> Ulcers, colitis, chronic diarrhea, bronchial asthma, atopic dermatitis, urticaria, angioneurotic edema, hay fever, arthritis, Raynaud's disease, hypertension, hyperthyroidism, amenorrhea, enuresis, paroxysmal tachycardia, migraines, impotence, general sexual dysfunctions, sleep-onset insomnia, alcoholism, and a full range of neurotic and psychotic disorders.

Stone Age Stress

Face it, stress is a reality in our day-to-day living and has always been with us, from the days of checking around corners for saber-toothed tigers, to living in a high-tech society in the twenty-first century. The only difference is how we respond to stress and how we perceive it.

I'm sure that if the experts were around in the Paleolithic Era, there would have been stress-related charts on the wall of every medicine man's cave, and food gathering in saber-toothed tiger-infested woods would probably have been on the top of the list.

We have always had problems, challenges, learning experiences, opportunities, obstacles, good times, bad times, and in-between times. That is what being human is all about and why we are here—to learn all we can and use the knowledge for our personal growth.

Stress is simply making problems out of
our learning experiences.

When we are under extreme stress, our body rebels to let us know we are not handling life in our best self-interest. What do we do then? Some people run to someone else to solve their problems or take chemicals, never figuring out what it was they were supposed to learn in the first place.

I read an article recently that stated the amount of money spent on tranquilizers each year in this country. Are you ready for this? Over $2 billion! Enough said.

Body Language

Let's talk about symptoms related to stress. A symptom can be anything from a headache to chronic diarrhea. Symptoms are the body's way of talking to us about the things we need to know about our body, what we need to change, and what we need to pay attention to. If we only tune in and listen to our body, it will tell us all we need to know to heal ourselves.

Many times, illnesses like diarrhea, nausea, and vomiting are the body's way of cleaning itself out. We seem to take in so many incompatible substances with our body chemistry, that eventually it must all go somewhere. Think of the air we breathe, the water we drink, the food we eat, and all of the chemicals in our environment. It is all taken into our body somehow; if not by direct means, then by indirect, such as absorption through the skin. The so-called "flu" is usually the body's way of cleaning out toxins. Be thankful the body has sense enough to do it for you.

A bout with the flu is the best time for rest and plenty of fluids; distilled water mixed with lemon juice is a good drink. Also, lactobacillus acidophilus (a "friendly" bacteria that can be purchased at health food stores) will replace any of the good bacteria in the lower bowel that may have been lost in the cleansing.

Other symptoms can tell us we are not taking good care of ourselves. Maybe we don't drink enough water, get enough sleep, or eat the right kinds of food. Many symptoms are the body's way of establishing balance and restoring health. In the case of an upper respiratory condition, a mild fever will inactivate many viruses, and mucus is produced to wash away the end products of the ongoing germ warfare. Coughing then blows the mucus out of the airways.

Over-the-Counter Stress

One of the biggest problems I see in society is the programming done by the media and medical community. We are programmed to think we should never experience discomfort of any kind and that having something like a fever is a bad thing. On the contrary, a fever is one of the body's defenses in fighting bacteria and viruses. A very high fever can certainly be destructive to body cells, but everyone is conditioned to squelch even the smallest hint of an elevated temperature.

Listen to the latest advertising pitches; they encourage you to take something for every little thing that might inconvenience you or cause discomfort. However, these may be symptoms of another problem and if we keep covering them up with our over-the-counter "quickie" reliefs, we may never get to the real cause. Many over-the-counter medications mask the messages the body is trying to send. Instead of giving in to immediate gratification and not wanting to be bothered by your body, stop and listen.

Take time to be in tune with yourself and correct even the smallest things before they get out of control.

I Can't Stress It Enough

It is my opinion that most of the stress we create for ourselves boils down to a self-love issue. When we have self-love, we are able to look at everything in our lives as something beautiful and rewarding. The concept of self-love does not mean being selfish or self-serving, and it does not mean you are better than anyone else. In case you haven't figured out the concept of self-love by now, here it is:

- You see yourself as a beautiful, wonderful person and everyone around you is equal.

- Not judging or condemning yourself or anyone else.

- Acceptance of self and others.

- Taking charge of your life and reaching for the highest growth and learning experiences possible.

- Loving the world around you and treating all that you encounter with respect and reverence.

- Enjoying the life you have chosen, living to the fullest, and making the changes you need without guilt or remorse.

- Knowing you deserve every bit of success that comes to you.

You don't have to learn a lot of complicated things, go to classes, or read many books to become a better person and have self-love. You just need to look around you and see all of the beautiful people and objects in your world.

It is, indeed, your world; you created it and everything in it. Love everything you see for the beauty it brings you and the lessons it allows you to learn.

The more you love, the more you have the capacity to love, and the more you are loved. It is the indisputable Law of Prosperity.

What you project to the world is
what you receive in return.

Life's Lessons

I always tell my daughter that if you choose to get angry or hurt in response to someone else's actions, look at what it is about them that gave you cause to be angry. First, consider whether or not you have exhibited some of that person's traits and whether or not you dislike those traits; or maybe they have problems you have already worked through and do not wish to slide back into. Either way, thank that person for teaching you a very valuable lesson and allowing you to grow that much more.

We are mirror images of each other.

Thanking that person and realizing the lesson you learned gives you a much better feeling about them than if you were to feed into their negativity. Always remember that everyone has their own lessons to learn and world to live in. They have also gotten themselves to where they are today.

Remember, we can all learn from each other. We are all teachers and students. We just need to tune in and become receptive.

The Illusion of Self-Control

One of the biggest problems many of us have is trying to control other people around us. This really can't be done and if you persist, things won't work out very well for either of you.

The concept of control is merely an illusion.

A good illustration is seed planting. When you plant a seed you can nurture and nourish and love it, but you cannot control it. You can't dictate its shape, size, color of leaves, or whether it will bear fruit or how much. If you use control over the growing plant (for example, pruning it as you would a bonsai tree), you stunt its growth and end up with a totally unnatural product. The same also applies to people. For many of us,

Allowing people to be themselves is one
of the hardest things to do.

In trying to control and manipulate, we create stress in others and ourselves. Yes, stress! You create stress for the other person, especially if they are trying to live up to your expectations, and you create stress for yourself by not allowing yourself to be natural and relaxed.

Great Expectations

Speaking of meeting expectations, here is a biggie! Somewhere along the trail of life, I was given a list of ten irrational thoughts. One I will never forget was, "I will be all things to all people at all times." The reason I will never forget this thought is because it is the one I needed to learn the most from. First of all, I needed to learn that I did not have to meet anyone's expectations but my own. Not those of my parents, boss, friends, or daughter. Next, I had to learn what was reasonable to expect from myself.

Catch a Goal

Goals are great to have and we wander aimlessly without them. However, goals need to be realistic and attainable by the person setting them. I like to set minor goals and major goals. The publication of this book was a *major* goal.

As with all goals, the key to attaining them is to take one step at a time and one day at a time. Don't bog yourself down with more than you can handle. When you do, you set yourself up for disappointment and things become stressful. If your minor goals are not accomplished in your set time frame, sit back and take a second look. Were the goals truly realistic for the time and place? Maybe they weren't. Be honest with yourself. Next, look at what you have accomplished and give yourself a pat on the back.

Always look at the positive aspects of your life. When I was a child, I remember hearing a song written by Irving Berlin that was about counting your blessings. The words in the song are just as applicable today as when they were written.

Have No Fear

Now let's talk about a big stress-maker—*fear.* Sprinkled throughout these pages, you will find little tidbits on fear and reasons for not accepting it and buying into it. Now we will talk about fear in the guise of stress. Even the word fear causes some people a tinge of stress. One of the best statements I've ever heard on fear was made by Franklin D. Roosevelt in 1933 during his inaugural address, "The only thing we have to fear is fear itself." As you can see, fear is very powerful and can conjure up every negative experience imaginable. We need to put fear in perspective and learn how to have control over it.

Laughter: The Best Medicine

One of the absolute best ways of dealing with fear is to laugh. See the humor in the situation and laugh out loud. Laughing is a release of tension in the body and mind. It alters your energy level and clears your head. Also, while you are laughing, you are unable to feed any fear into the situation.

Remember, thoughts are things, and whatever we think, we can manifest. It has been said many times by many people that laughter is the best medicine. Think about how good you feel when you have had a good laugh. Recapture that feeling whenever you need it, for that is why we have memory banks. Let the happy joyous feeling spread throughout your entire body. Feel it and enjoy it.

Silver Linings

Don't buy into anyone's preconceived notion of how you *should* react to a situation. In fact, you will really benefit from getting rid of all of your "shoulds," "oughts," and "musts." For instance, if you have lost your job and everyone wants to feel bad for you, don't let them and don't you do it either. Instead of dwelling on the loss, look at the opportunity of the situation. Ask yourself what you want to do with your life. What do you *really* want to do with your life?

If you sit around and worry about the situation, it certainly can't get any better. However, if you truly believe that everything happens for the best possible reason or learning experience and your needs will be provided for, you can look at this as a positive experience.

When I first put a loved one in a drug treatment program, I knew it was going to be a long haul and I had absolutely no idea how I was going to pay for it; but I knew it was the right thing to do. In the end, everything worked out fine. We never went hungry, there was always a roof over our heads, and I found that I had the most wonderful, supportive friends in the world. I never programmed the experience for failure, only for success. People will say to me, "Oh, what a horrible experience you had to go through!" I don't look at it that way. It was not easy, but I learned so much and met so many wonderful people that, yes, I would go through it again.

We are here to learn from our experiences,
but we don't have to keep them.

Learn what you need to learn from a situation
and get on with your life.

9

....

Food for Thought

IN DOING THE mountains of research necessary for this chapter, it became clear that most nutrition experts have valid points to make and many statistics and anecdotes to back them up. These experts tell stories of foods, herbs, and remedies that have worked for them and their clients. There is tremendous diversity in their approaches and conclusions to nutrition. The one conclusion I have come to is one I have supported for everything in my life:

If you believe in it, it will work for you!

Food has always been one of my first loves, and I received a great deal of pleasure from writing this chapter on nutrition; but this chapter, as with the others, is not cast in stone. It is a guide to better nourishment of the body shell that carries us around in this life. I encourage you to enjoy every second of your life to the fullest, and that means mealtime too. Food is something to enjoy. We as humans must eat, so why not eat what we enjoy and at the same time, know that we are nourishing our bodies? Savor the things in your life to the fullest!

The Good, the Bad, and You

When it comes to food, I believe there is no good food or bad food. The question is: What is good for you as an individual? Our beliefs are formed early in our childhood through the influence of our family and the media. When we put labels on food and subscribe to a "good food/bad food" belief system, there will be a conflict. The food we consider "bad" will not nourish us because we have labeled it as such. Some people believe that all food they enjoy is good for them and nourishes their body—yes, including chocolate! Your belief system may allow you to eat ten cookies without weight gain, or it may only allow you to eat two. What are your beliefs about food?

If you believe your body will use what it needs from the food you eat and eliminate what it doesn't, then that belief system will work for you. There is wholesomeness and loving life force in everything we eat. Each of us is a separate entity, different and unique, and what is good for one person may not be good for another.

It is the response of your mind and
body to a food that matters.

Ideally Yours

Affirm your health and fitness. Do not say you are losing weight because your subconscious will actually think it has lost something and will try to find it again. Affirm the reconstructing of your body image to a much slimmer you. Confirm your ideal weight, but let's be reasonable with this, folks. Pick a weight that you feel comfortable with, not one that is right for someone else of a different body build. Also, do not aspire to weigh what someone else thinks is right for you.

Advertising shows the "perfect" body as slightly anorexic. How many of us have that perfect body? I know I don't, nor do I want it. My life is not tied up in someone else's body image. Part of loving my body also means accepting its image. If you feel you must have another body image and need a model, instead of looking at magazines or television, go to the grocery store or mall and pick out a model that is ideally yours.

Why Do You Eat?

Today, many people go through all the craziness of crash diets, exercise programs, and the yo-yo syndrome of taking weight off and putting it back on. In reality, most people never discover the real reasons for their struggle with body weight. Many use food for the same reason they would use drugs or alcohol—to push down their feelings. Food then becomes a destructive force in their lives. Our food is meant to nourish our bodies with loving care, not to destroy or harm them.

If you feel that part of taking responsibility for your health is eating natural foods, cutting down on fats, and increasing your exercise, that belief system will work for you.

Think healthy and trim.

We create our own reality. Believe in yourself and know that you create "you" and are responsible for "you." Anytime you place negative vibrations into food, such as "I know this is not good for me," you get what you ask for. If you say, "This is fattening," of course it is fattening! You thought it and created it.

Individual Beliefs

The following information in this chapter is merely a guideline for an alternative-eating lifestyle. Yes, it is possible to eat what you want and remain healthy, but what you want to eat must correspond with what you believe is healthy for you. Most people believe junk food is not healthy for them and they are a bad person for eating it. The body translates this thought into "bad" nutrition. If your belief system determines your nutritional habits and you believe in a lighter dietary style, that's what will work for you. The following information on junk food, fats, and sugars are good guidelines for that belief system.

Fast Food and Junk Food

As most of us know, the picture-perfect hamburger, brimming with juices and fresh vegetables, is not the one that gets wrapped in paper and shoved under a heat lamp at the local fast food place. These "whole-beef patties" get anywhere from 38 to 56 percent of their calories from fat. By any standards, that is a lot of fat. Many times, the vegetables have been prepared far in advance, thus losing valuable vitamins with every minute they sit, To top it off, the white flour bun that houses the burger has virtually no fiber and minimal nutrition.

We are constantly bombarded by fast food advertisements. They tell us how great certain foods taste, but they don't tell us they are also loaded with fats, salt, and sugar. I once saw an advertisement placed by a local fast food chain for their new chicken sandwich. This was an attempt to capitalize on the move away from red meat. The poor piece of chicken had been breaded with a batter, deep-fried, and shoved into a refined flour bun which was saturated with mayonnaise. Whatever nutrition might have been left in the chicken certainly was neutralized by all of that fat.

Fast foods are notorious for their high salt, sugar, and fat content. They are also low in potassium, fiber, and essential vitamins and minerals, and most nutrients are processed out. Many popular high-calorie foods on the market are also some of the most processed. They include white bread, rolls, crackers, donuts, cookies, cakes, alcohol, whole milk, beef, and soft drinks.

Processing foods robs them not only of the vital life force they pass on to us, but of their essential nutrients as well. Some of these nutrients are replaced artificially, but studies are finding that these are not as easily assimilated by the body as those from natural foods. We are still cut short on vital nourishment.

Many fast food restaurants now have salad bars in their effort to meet the new public demand for healthier food. This gives you the option of controlling the amount of fat in your meal. Since salad bars present choices, it becomes your responsibility to choose what is best for your body.

In the last forty years, Americans have increased their soft drink intake by 80 percent and their junk food intake by 85 percent. At the same time, they are eating fewer dairy products, fresh fruits, and vegetables. If you want to know just how popular fast, junk, and snack foods are, watch an hour of television, pick up a magazine, or look at other forms of advertising.

A good way to cut down on junk food and sugars is simply to not buy them. If they are not in the house, you and your family will not eat them. Be firm. If there are those in your family who have to have junk food, let them get it themselves. Make everyone in your family responsible for their own health.

Instead of snacks like potato chips or candy, try raw fruits and vegetables or unsalted and unbuttered popcorn.

I have heard comments that "naked" popcorn tastes a lot like packing peanuts. I am more into the texture of the food, so I enjoy it plain—the buttered variety now tastes too greasy for me.

The Sugar Story

When we eat excess sugar, we become deficient in valuable vitamins and minerals because sugar tends to dull our appetite for other foods. The average American eats about 120 pounds of sugar a year, and most is hidden in the processed and fast foods we eat.

Some conditions associated with refined sugars are tooth decay, obesity, heart problems, and maturity-onset diabetes. If you must eat sugar, fructose (the natural sugar derived from fruit) is a better choice for you. It is less likely to cause cavities and does not need as much insulin to move from the blood to the body cell. Fructose can be found in health food stores, usually in a powdered form. Experiment using fructose in your recipes in place of sugar. Other alternatives are honey, barley malt, molasses, and maple syrup. The body absorbs these natural sugars more slowly than refined sugars and does not experience a sugar jolt (the rapid high associated with the infusion of sugar, which is followed by a fast drop when the sugar is exhausted from the system).

Helpful Hints

Here are some suggestions for cutting back on the amount of sugar in your diet:

- Cut the sugar in fruit juices by mixing them with one-half water or mineral water. Do not use carbonated water, as the phosphorus may block the absorption of iron into the blood stream.

- If you cut down on sugar gradually, your family may never know the difference. Instead of one cup of sugar in a recipe, use ⅔ cup. Use more fruit in your desserts and try desserts of just fruit and cheese.

- Try sparkling mineral waters instead of soda.

- If you drink alcohol, lighten it up with equal amounts of mineral water. This will cut the alcohol and calories in half.

- Make your own peanut butter or other nut butters without using sugar or salt.

- Instead of sugar, use spices, flavorings, liqueurs, low-calorie maple syrup, and fruit juices.

- Eat dried fruits for snacks. They are rich in iron, copper, and potassium. The sugar is more concentrated in dried fruits but, again, it is fructose and metabolizes differently.

- Use unsweetened cocoa instead of chocolate.

- Be creative with the natural sugar of fruits instead of refined sugar. For example, use sweet apples and a combination of spices in an apple pie. Omit the refined sugar. Use orange juice and grated orange rind in your pie crust to perk up your fruit pies.

The key words here are: *Be creative!*

The Fats of Life

While researching this project, I discovered a lot of disagreement among experts on the subject of polyunsaturated fats. I finally came to the conclusion that there is no proof that eating unsaturated fats, as opposed to saturated fats, will prevent heart attacks. There are still too many other factors involved.

Another "fat" argument today is the lecithin issue. Lecithin is a compound that has the ability to dissolve cholesterol and other fats. The controversial egg yolk not only contains cholesterol, but lecithin too. I believe in the benefits of lecithin and think that Mother Nature uses her own system of checks and balances and this is one of them. We merely have to accept it as such.

One of the brightest discoveries along the line of natural, preventative health is Omega 3 fatty acids. These acids are found in fatty, northern ocean fish and have many beneficial properties for us. They lower cholesterol and triglyceride levels, and reduce the tendency of blood to form clots in the blood vessels. The acids also help to improve development in infants who are being breast-fed, and reduce arthritic inflammation and the risk of some cancers.

Fish that are highest in Omega 3 acids are anchovies, salmon, sardines, shad, albacore, and blue-fin tuna. Fish with a medium amount of Omega 3 acids include catfish, pacific halibut, swordfish, and trout. Fish with the lowest amounts of Omega 3 acids are cod, flounder, haddock, pike, red snapper, sea bass, and whiting.

In order to maintain the balance of nutrients in our diets, we should get 30 percent of our total calories from fats. We need fats for several reasons. Fats are needed to absorb vitamins A, D, E, and K, and for storage areas in our body. There are certain parts of our body that are protected from injury by the fatty pads which surround them. Fats also give our face its features.

Calculating Fat

Here is an easy formula to calculate the total amount of calories you are getting from fat. A gram of fat has nine calories, while a gram of protein or carbohydrate has four. Take the grams of fat in a food serving and multiply it by nine to get the number of calories in the fat. Then, divide the fat calories by the total calories to get the percentage of calories you get from fat. The healthiest percentage of fat calories is 30 percent; therefore, your daily requirement is forty to eighty grams of fat.

Helpful Hints

Here are a few helpful hints for reducing the amount of fat in your diet. Try them with an open mind and you may find you like the lighter taste better. Often, once you get used to a lighter version of food, the heavier fats seem much too greasy.

- There are many fat-free products on the market that you can try in your cooking. Some make great substitutes, while others taste terrible. You will have to experiment and find the ones you prefer.

- Vegetable cream soups made from scratch can be made without cream. Use starchy vegetables, like potatoes or carrots, and purée to a very smooth consistency. Mix them with skim milk and add seasonings, such as parsley, sage, rosemary, or thyme.

- Trim all visible traces of fat off your red meat.

- Let your soups and stews sit in the refrigerator overnight and then skim off the fat. Sitting overnight allows the ingredients to mingle and will meld the flavors.

- Remove all fat and skin from poultry before cooking. If you choose to leave your chicken unskinned for the flavor it gives during cooking, don't eat the skin.

- Use light oils—olive, corn, or safflower.

- Use part-skim milk cheeses instead of whole milk cheeses.

- Buttermilk is lower in fat than whole milk and is a good substitute in baking.

- Instead of sour cream on your baked potato, purée one part nonfat buttermilk and four parts lowfat cottage cheese together. Plain yogurt is also good to use.

- Cook rice, pasta, and vegetables without salt or fat. Use lowfat sauces or seasonings to give them flavor.

- Lowfat yogurt can be used as a substitute for eggs and oils in some baking.

The Prune Factor

Puréed prunes are now being used in baking in place of fat. One serving (ten prunes) has 6.6 grams of fiber, less than one gram of fat, is high in potassium and beta-carotene, has diphenylisatin (a natural laxative), and is high in pectin. Pectin helps form a film around the air in baked goods in the same way that butter or shortening does. It also traps and enhances flavor. Prunes are high in sorbitol, a humectant that attracts and binds moisture and enhances shelf life. Lekvar (a sweet pastry filling made of prunes or apricots) can be used as a one-to-one substitute, or you can purée your own (six ounces of prunes with six tablespoons of hot water in a food processor makes one cup). Be sure to soak the prunes in the hot water first before puréeing. Some products I have had success with are chocolate chip cookies, brownies, gingersnaps, muffins, and quickbreads.

Designer Labels

How can you know what you are eating? Read the labels. The primary ingredient is listed first, with the rest following in descending order. When reading bread labels, look for the word "whole." This denotes a whole grain rather than one where the germ and bran have been milled away.

MSG, or monosodium glutamate, is a flavor-enhancing chemical that many people are sensitive to. It comes in numerous processed foods such as frozen vegetables. If you do not want MSG in your frozen veggies, freeze them yourself. Dip them in boiling water for one minute with just a tiny bit of salt. The potassium in the food will counteract the salt. Do not add extra salt in cooking. Fresh is always best when it comes to your nutrition. If you must use canned vegetables, rinse off the sodium before cooking them.

Nitrates are another group of chemicals that are used in processed foods. They are mainly used in cured meats. Many people are now finding that some of their allergies are from the nitrates in foods. To counteract the negative effects of nitrates, drink orange juice or eat fruits that are high in vitamin C.

Cholesterol Is Not an Ugly Word

Cholesterol is found in many of the foods we eat and is a substance necessary for the health of body tissues. Our bodies also produce certain amounts of cholesterol. Cholesterol is used in the formation of estrogen, testosterone, adrenal hormones, and nerve tissue, and it is used in metabolizing vitamin D and bile (an internal chemical necessary for the digestion of fats). As you can see, cholesterol is a very important part of our daily requirements. If we do not ingest enough cholesterol, our bodies will make it for us.

If you have a problem with blocking things in your life, such as relationships or feelings, you may have a tendency to eat foods that put physical blocks into your body. These blocks may be made from cholesterol and fats.

Cholesterol can stick to the walls of your arteries and veins, causing rough surfaces. As the blood flows through your blood vessels, fats and blood cells stick to these rough surfaces and build up little barricades. Eventually, this build-up can clog an entire blood vessel. Clogged blood vessels anywhere in the body are not conducive to good health.

Another instance in which our bodies produce excess cholesterol is our reaction to stress. When we allow ourselves to get easily upset, we tend to stay in an agitated mode. Any type of prolonged emotional upheaval, whether it is released or held inside, will cause the gall bladder to produce cholesterol and pour it into the system to be circulated around the body. Here again, our physical health depends on our mental health. Without question, our minds are very powerful and can generate a destructive or a healing force, whichever we choose.

No Passing on the Carbs

Carbohydrates are the main source of energy in the body. When not being used for energy, they are converted to fat and stored in the body for energy at a later date. Carbohydrates should make up 50 percent of our daily intake of food.

Complex carbohydrates are superior to simple sugars. Simple sugar molecules are immediately metabolized and will produce a sugar rush. The complex carbohydrates are made of complex chemical chains that break down at a much slower, controlled rate and release energy at a more even pace. These carbohydrates are found in whole natural foods, not refined foods. Some examples of whole natural foods are whole grains, rice, whole-grain breads, pasta, beans, potatoes, and many other vegetables and fruits.

Going with the Grain

Grains are probably the most versatile of the complex carbohydrates. They are a natural energy source and very rich in fiber. Whole grains, with their high natural-fiber content, help protect against heart disease. They are also a storehouse of nutrition. There are three parts of the grain with different nutritional values:

Germ: the tiny heart of the seed that contains vitamins, oils, protein, and vitamin E.

Endosperm: the starchy bulk that nourishes the germ and contains starch and protein.

Bran: the tough covering that protects the seed and contains minerals, fiber, protein, and some B vitamins.

Rice is one of the most popular grains used around the world as a nutritional staple. If you are depending on rice for a large part of the protein in your diet, polished white rice is your best bet. The protein in polished rice is more available to the body than that in brown rice, but make sure that you get plenty of the B vitamins that are lost from polished rice, such as riboflavin, niacin, pyridoxine, and thiamine. Please refer to the vitamin section of this chapter for more information on what foods contain vitamin B.

When I bake, I like to use different grains for variety; I use whole wheat, oats, barley, rye, millet, buckwheat, blue corn, rice, soy, and triticale. If you like, you can even mix some of these flours to explore a whole new world in baking.

Protein

Protein is important for tissue growth and repair, since every cell in our body is built on a protein structure. Twenty percent of our diet should be protein. There are basically two types of protein used by the body: vegetable and animal. Vegetable protein is high in complex carbohydrates and fiber, and low in fat. These nutrients help lower cholesterol levels in the blood. Dried beans and peas contain up to 20 to 25 percent of this type of protein.

The other type of protein comes from animals. Animal proteins that are lowest in fat are fish, shellfish, skinless chicken or turkey, lowfat dairy products, and lowfat cuts of meat. Animal protein contains a better balance of amino acids, which are the building blocks of protein. Our bodies are capable of making all but eight of the twenty amino acids used to make protein; therefore, these eight must be obtained from the food we eat. They are called "essential" amino acids because they are essential for protein production.

Vegetables and grains alone provide only part of the essential amino acids, but they can be combined to form the complete amino acids. Grains are low in lysine and high in methionine, while beans are high in lysine and low in methionine. Dried peas, beans, and peanuts are the richest source of vegetable protein. Recommended grains are rice, wheat, corn, barley, oats, and seeds. The ideal ratio is one part legume (dried beans or peas) to two parts grains. Oats are higher in protein than any other grain and the easiest to prepare. They can be cooked as cereals, used in salads, or sprinkled over food.

Let's Not Cause a Big Stink

Many people experience gas problems from eating dried beans. The gases are formed as a by-product of digestion. There are ways to reduce or eliminate the gas-forming chemicals of beans. Many seasonings and fats used in preparing bean dishes aid in the digestive process, thus helping to eliminate the gas problem. Some of these seasonings are cumin, coriander, and asafoetida. Another hint is to soak the beans twice and discard the water each time. I follow this procedure when I make my beans from scratch and never have any digestive problems.

Veggies versus Meat

There has been and probably always will be a great deal of controversy between vegetarians and nonvegetarians. I, for one, started becoming uncomfortable with red meat years ago. I stopped eating red meat because I did not agree with the conditions and treatment of the animals in the slaughterhouses. For me, this was hard to digest, thus making meat physically indigestible.

People who consistently eat little or no meat tend to have fewer incidences of cancer, heart disease, high blood pressure, and osteoporosis. Some vegetarians felt they had fewer headaches and were mentally more alert after eliminating meat from their diets.

For some people, red meat is nourishing. If you do eat red meat, use the leaner cuts to cut down on the fat content. Leaner cuts include round steak, round roast, sirloin, flank steak, ham steak, pork loin chops, lamb leg, loin chops, veal steak, veal chops, and veal cutlets. I use turkey breast or thighs instead of beef or pork in my recipes. Ground turkey can also be used in place of ground beef in dishes like chili and spaghetti. I am creative with my seasonings and think the taste is even better than that of red meat.

Turkey is a very versatile and nutritious form of protein. It contains B vitamins, iron, zinc, and other trace minerals. When you trim the skin off turkey, it is lower in fat than chicken. It also has 50 percent less fat than ground beef.

Soy to the World

The soybean has very high-quality protein and is low in cholesterol and triglycerides. Its versatility is demonstrated in dairy products, tofu, and even soy burgers. Fields of soybean can produce up to twenty times more protein than the same fields used to feed cattle.

Tofu is a soy product that has been used in Asia for many years as a quality source of protein, but is just now starting to gain in popularity in the Western cultures. Tofu is very high in vegetable protein, calcium, and iron, and has minimal fat, no cholesterol, and only a trace of sodium. Not having much taste of its own, tofu will pick up the taste of whatever you prepare it with. I like to mix it in my tuna salad for sandwiches. It increases the volume and nutrition of the mixture and everyone thinks it's chopped egg white.

There are virtually endless ways of using tofu in your diet. You can use it in salad dressings, dips, or mashed as a spread. A great salad dressing is tofu, salad oil, lemon juice, herbs, and spices whirled in a blender. Tofu can be fried, made into burgers, scrambled with veggies, or cubed in a broth. It can serve as a replacement for cheese in baked dishes and is great to use in desserts. Tofu can be found in any large grocery store.

Say Cheese

Dairy products also contain protein. Here are some interesting healing facts on two dairy products: cheese and yogurt. Cheese helps protect your teeth by stimulating saliva flow. It also inhibits acid production, which eats away at tooth enamel. Some of the most protective cheeses are aged cheddar, Monterey Jack, and Swiss.

Yogurt is perfect for restoring the bacterial flora in the intestines, especially after a bout with diarrhea. If you are taking antibiotics, it is a good idea to eat a lot of yogurt. Why? Because many antibiotics kill the natural bacteria found in the bowel; the live cultures in the yogurt help restore the natural bacteria. Yogurt can also help heal cold sores and lower cholesterol levels. When buying yogurt, look for the kind with live bacteria cultures.

Fiber

Before the twentieth century, average people ate a large amount of plant-based fiber. It is the lack of adequate fiber in our diets that now help precipitate "civilized" illnesses, including heart conditions, bowel diseases, and gall bladder problems.

No Holding Back

Today, modern man eats an abundance of refined foods. A diet rich in these foods can lead to problems like constipation or the elimination of a hard, small stool. Being constipated leads to straining and increased pressure inside the body. This pressure can cause a hernia, hemorrhoids, varicose veins, and diverticulitis (inflammation of the large bowel).

Holding stool inside the body traps certain cancer-causing toxins. These toxins, even if they do not cause cancer, are disruptive to the entire body, especially the brain. Holding stool can also cause the breeding of unnatural bacteria inside the intestinal tract, which causes inflammation of the intestinal tissue. I have heard it said that after the age of sixty, "The sun rises and sets on your bowels." Well, it doesn't have to be that way with an adequate amount of fiber in your diet and a change in your thought process. Look to see where you may be holding something back in your life.

Bran Overboard

For a period of time, many people jumped on the "bran" bandwagon with some disastrous results. Some people were ingesting large amounts of bran with very little water, which helps the bulk through the large intestine. The result of a lot of bran and a small amount of fluid is a concrete-like substance in the lower bowel that may need to be surgically removed. Just adding fiber to your diet in the form of bran will not give you all of the desired results. You need to include the whole grain so that all of its components can work together as nature intended.

That's Psylly

One of the most useful fibers in our food is pectin. It is found in many of the edible parts of fruits and vegetables. Apples have an abundance of pectin and dried apples have concentrated pectin. Anyone who has ever canned jams or jellies is familiar with its gelling qualities. In the intestinal tract, pectin absorbs water and helps make the stool bulky and soft. Another of pectin's endearing qualities is its binding power with many toxic chemicals, such as cyclamates. It carries them harmlessly out of the body in the stool.

Another natural fiber used as a laxative is psyllium seed husks. Its ability to absorb large amounts of water makes it good for constipation as well as diarrhea. In the case of constipation, it adds moisture to a dry, hard stool. During a bout of diarrhea, it absorbs the excess water in a liquid stool. Psyllium seed husks can be found in most health food stores.

Life is Roughage

There are two main types of fiber: insoluble and soluble. Insoluble fiber helps foods pass through the intestine; soluble fiber causes a slow rise in blood sugar and an even distribution of energy, and aids in lowering cholesterol levels. Soluble fiber also forms a gel that binds with cholesterol and passes out of the body.

Dried beans are one of our best sources of fiber, as they have minimal fat and no cholesterol. Brown rice has three times more fiber than white rice. It also contains more B vitamins, iron, magnesium, and zinc. To take advantage of the added nutrition in high-fiber foods, you should have smaller portions of meat and larger portions of grains and vegetables in your dishes. By the way, for you "meat and potatoes" people, all kinds of potatoes are very high in fiber; it is what you put on them that can be fattening.

Other vegetables high in fiber are mushrooms, celery, and the whole cabbage family, including cauliflower, broccoli, brussels sprouts, collard greens, and kohlrabi. These vegetables also contain sulforphane, which is known to enhance the cell's ability to protect itself from cancer.

Substitute whole-grain recipes in baking. In processed white flour, 80 percent of the nutrients are lost and usually only four of them—thiamine, riboflavin, niacin, and iron—are replaced. There are many different whole-grain flours on the market now. Try something different and experiment!

There are many ready-made baked goods on the shelves with whole grain ingredients. If you are looking for a high-fiber, lowfat snack, instead of a bagel with cream cheese, have a whole-wheat bagel with Neufchâtel cheese.

Keep It Regular

Another important aspect of regular elimination is exercise. Regular exercise helps tone all of the muscles in our body, including the internal ones. The intestinal tract is just one big muscle. To continue working properly, it must remain healthy and be in good shape. The movement of our body gives our internal organs a type of internal massage. Drinking an adequate amount of fluids not only keeps our body hydrated, but also helps to keep the stool soft and moist. As part of the body's survival system, water is reabsorbed back into the body from the large intestine.

When we do not drink enough water, the body feels it has to reabsorb every ounce it can get. It does this by pulling fluid out of the stool mass, thus making it very dry and hard, which leads to constipation. Water also helps to cleanse the body from the inside out. The addition of lemon juice aids the liver in its detoxifying qualities.

Don't Give It Up

As you are reading this, you are probably thinking about making some changes in your eating lifestyle. Everything in moderation is key here, since our bodies can usually handle most anything this way. As long as we are talking about minimizing certain foods in your diet, here is a helpful hint on how to do it successfully: It isn't necessary to completely give up a food. Instead of denying yourself, savor every second of the experience and soon it will take less and less to satisfy you.

When working on reducing your body size, the preceding tips work very well. You should also keep in mind other factors, such as eating regular meals. When you skip meals, especially breakfast and lunch, you are usually hungrier later and may overeat.

Daily exercise helps keep your metabolism revved up and at an even pace. An even metabolism burns more calories without giving you highs and lows in your energy levels. You are also less likely to get a midafternoon slump.

Food on My Mind

There are many other factors that involve our eating habits. Hormones and their cycles affect many women's appetites. Ten days after a woman ovulates there is an increase in progesterone and a decrease in estrogen in her body. This change in hormone levels sparks an increase in appetite and causes many women to take in more fat, sugar, and salt. These substances help contribute to the symptoms of Premenstrual Syndrome, more commonly known as PMS. To help alleviate most PMS symptoms, eat more grains and raw fresh vegetables during the latter half of the menstrual cycle.

Foods also affect the chemicals in our brains. Eating pure carbohydrates, like fruit and pasta, stimulate a chemical in the brain known as serotonin. Serotonin has a calming effect and helps us sleep. Eating pure carbohydrates without protein causes drowsiness. On the other hand, eating foods that are high in protein increases alertness.

Eating pure lecithin, found in egg yolks, organ, and other meats, may raise the level of a chemical known as acetylcholine in the brain. Some studies show that increased levels of acetylcholine help us to remember.

Distress interferes with the parasympathetic nervous system that controls our digestive process. This process includes hydrochloric acid secretion, and pancreas, digestive enzymes, liver, and bile secretions. When something interferes with this system, your food is not digested properly. Next, fats and toxins from the inadequate metabolism of food back up in your system and you end up with gas, bloating, and heartburn. One of the unpleasant side effects of eating or drinking too fast is the hiccups. The hiccups momentarily paralyze the esophagus to slow us down. It is a protective mechanism.

Vitamins and Minerals

The food we eat consists mainly of protein, fat, and carbohydrate, and there is a very small percent (approximately 2 percent) of food substances that we cannot live without—vitamins and minerals. These chemicals are vital to a well-nourished body. They help convert the foods we eat into energy, and are necessary for regulating the electrical activity in our nervous system and maintaining healthy skin.

Many drugs deplete the body of vitamins and minerals. Aspirin depletes vitamin C and diuretics wash out a variety of different minerals. If you are going to be on any drug for a period of time, ask your doctor or counselor what foods you will need to supplement your diet.

Alcohol will also deplete the body of vitamins very fast. The commercial processing of citrus fruits destroys at least 30 percent of the usable vitamin C. Fruits and vegetables are best eaten raw or slightly cooked. Here are some cooking and preparation tips for conserving your vitamins and minerals:

- When preparing fruits and vegetables, do not remove edible peels or soak them. Do minimal chopping and do it immediately before cooking. An exposed surface will cause dissipation of valuable vitamins and minerals.

- Defrost frozen foods in the refrigerator and use their juices. The juices will contain many of the vitamins and minerals.

Precious Minerals

Calcium: It is well-known that calcium is the foundation of our skeletal structure. What many people do not know is that calcium helps to keep our blood pressure normal and protects against colon cancer. It is now known that the protective effects of calcium in dairy products override the sodium and cholesterol. Dairy foods also have vitamin D, which helps us absorb the calcium. Look for this in the "fortified" foods. Calcium without vitamin D is of little use to the body. For those concerned with osteoporosis, vigorous exercise three times a week will help the bones reabsorb the calcium from the blood stream.

Rich sources of calcium are dairy products, green leafy vegetables, parsley, broccoli, beans, tofu, and canned salmon with the bones.

Copper: Diets low in copper can lead to cholesterol elevation.

Foods that contain copper are organ meats, legumes, grains, oysters, and other shellfish.

Iron: Iron is needed for the production of red blood cells. It is the element that carries the oxygen in our blood to the body tissues. Also, there is a possibility that children with an iron deficiency have a greater tendency to absorb lead, which can lead to lead poisoning. To help absorb the iron in vegetables, eat them with vitamin C, which is found in tomatoes, red peppers, and potatoes. Eating a little meat, fish, or chicken will also help.

Foods rich in iron are red meat, fish, poultry, seeds, beans, broccoli, leafy greens, tofu, apricots, and raisins.

Potassium: Many people are not aware that potassium will help balance some of the harmful effects of excess sodium in the body. Again, we see that nature has its own checks and balances. Salt substitutes, which are made from potassium, are not the best choice for those who secrete excess potassium—people with impaired kidneys or diabetes, and elderly people taking non-steroidal, anti-inflammatory medication. Sodium is needed in the body. Together, sodium and potassium help regulate the heartbeat, body fluids, and electrical activity.

Foods high in potassium are melons, bananas, citrus fruits and juices, potatoes, dried peas and beans, tomatoes, dried fruits, carrots, mushrooms, apricots, watermelon, rhubarb, and all varieties of greens.

Trace elements: These are very small, but very essential minerals. Trace elements help keep the immune system intact, regulate blood pressure, and reduce cholesterol in the blood. Several of the minerals are zinc, copper, magnesium, chromium, and selenium.

Trace elements are found in most fruits and vegetables.

Zinc: A lack of zinc in your diet can cause your taste buds to malfunction, and foods may not be as enjoyable as they used to be. In older people, a lack of zinc appears to produce a cycle of lack of appetite and poor nutrition.

Foods high in zinc are oysters, fish, green beans, lima beans, nuts, and whole grains.

The ABCs

Vitamin A: Vitamin A is essential for many reasons, including vision, healthy skin, and resistance to infection. Beta-carotene, which forms vitamin A in the body, helps protect cells from free radicals. Lycopene is another carotenoid found to be even better at trapping free radicals than beta-carotene. It is the red pigment found in tomatoes, red peppers, pink grapefruit, and watermelons.

Foods high in vitamin A and beta-carotene are all greens, carrots, red peppers, apricots, cantaloupes, mangos, fresh beans, and peas.

The B vitamins: There are several B vitamins on which whole books have been written. B vitamins are necessary for the function and maintenance of just about every part and organ of the body. A good example is folic acid. Folic acid helps to regulate cell growth. Low levels of folate are found in some older adults with senile-type behavior. Vitamin B_{12} deficiency, which is associated with aging, may be due to a low production of stomach acid. This causes bacteria in the stomach to use the B_{12} for its own use. Vitamin deficiencies may also go hand in hand with some of the negative attitudes associated with aging.

Foods rich in the B vitamins are asparagus, bananas, brans, broccoli, brussels sprouts, cabbage, cantaloupes, corn on the cob, cottage cheese, dried beans, peas, liver, orange juice, romaine lettuce, raw spinach, raisins, mushrooms, yeast breads, and yogurt.

Vitamin C: Healthy skin, gums, and prevention of the common cold are usually associated with vitamin C. This vitamin is also very important for blood clotting. Sprouts are very high in vitamin C. They have 12 percent more protein than the seeds they come from, three to ten times more vitamin B, and are very high in vitamins A, E, and K. They have a significant amount of chlorophyll in their leaves. Best of all, sprouts can be grown organically in your home. Seeds good for sprouting are beans, peas, alfalfa, wheat, rye, oats, barley, mung beans, radish, sunflower, soy, and fenugreek.

In addition to sprouts, foods high in vitamin C are leafy greens, red peppers, citrus fruits, kiwi fruit, apricots, potatoes, cauliflower, asparagus, and fresh peas and beans.

Vitamin D: This vitamin strengthens bones and teeth and is necessary for the heart, nerves, and the thyroid gland.

Foods rich in vitamin D are egg yolks, liver, and milk.

Vitamin E: Vitamin E is one of the essential components of cell walls, especially in the heart and lungs. Smokers should always supplement their diets with vitamin E.

Foods rich in vitamin E are dark green vegetables, fruits, and nuts.

Vitamin K: This vitamin is essential for the coagulation or clotting of blood.

Foods rich in vitamin K are leafy green vegetables, beef liver, yogurt, and oatmeal.

Healing Foods

For hundreds of years, before the advent of modern medicine, herbs and foods were used for healing. Even today, many people still rely on the natural healing powers given to us by Mother Nature. For many, these remedies work even better than chemical medicines. Natural foods do not interfere with the body's natural immune system and do not have disruptive side effects. Working with these foods is also a part of the very important process of taking responsibility for one's health. When we take that initiative of self-responsibility, we give our body a very powerful message. It is a message of self-healing and it can put into motion many of the body's own healing actions. Some of the more common foods used for maintaining health are listed.

Apples: Apples are often used as a laxative because they have a purging effect on the body. There are certain chemicals found naturally in apples that help the body rid itself of toxins. These toxins may accumulate in our bodies from our environment and from the foods we eat. Asians use apples for cleansing the liver, colon, spleen, and kidneys. Eating raw apples will also reduce plaque on your teeth. Apples are also a good source of boron, which may help prevent calcium leakage from the bones. For a total body cleansing, Edgar Cayce, author of books on natural healing, recommends a three-day diet of apples followed by two tablespoons of olive oil on the last day. I tried it once, and I must say that I did feel cleaned out.

Apricots: These beautiful fruits are a wonderful source of beta-carotene.

Blueberries: Many people have used blueberries to successfully treat diarrhea. Blackberries also have many of the same antidiarrheal properties.

Beets: For anyone with liver problems, beets will help cleanse the toxins filtered in the liver. These toxins may come from medicines, air, or processed food.

Cabbage: This plant has been used by healers for centuries. Today, many people use fresh-pressed juice as a treatment for stomach ulcers. Cabbage is also a great source of fiber.

Cauliflower: This vegetable causes an increase in enzyme activity, which helps clean the body of chemical pollutants.

Cherries: Eaten daily, cherries have been know to relieve the pain of gout.

Chlorophyll: This is the lifeblood of the plant and is very useful for people too. You can drink it or use it topically. Chlorophyll can aid in healing skin problems and has some cancer-fighting properties. For many people, it is a digestive aid and fights tooth decay. Many women also use it as a douche for trichomonas, a vaginal infection.

Chocolate: Chocolate lovers are going to love this—chocolate contains a substance that can be used to stimulate the kidneys to excrete more fluid from the body. It has also been used to relax smooth muscle tissue in people with asthma, enabling them to breathe easier.

Corn: Corn silk tea is used as a diuretic; by many in Europe and Asia it is used for bladder and kidney problems.

Cranberries: The juice and berries of this fruit are now a medically accepted aid for people with chronic bladder and kidney problems. They can also be used as a local application for the treatment of hemorrhoids.

Cucumbers: Just recently it was discovered that cucumbers have an enzyme that helps cholesterol pass quickly through the body without being absorbed.

Garlic: Garlic is not only one of my favorite seasonings, but one of the most versatile of the healing foods. It can be taken for everything from high blood pressure to infections. Garlic has been a staple in Oriental medicine for thousands of years. It is used as a diuretic, a substance that promotes urination, and relieves simple edema. Garlic is also used as an energy tonic and antibiotic.

Alliin is a substance found in the garlic bulb that, when ground down, becomes allicin, a powerful antibiotic agent. Used in this way, it does not upset the body's own immune system as many man-made antibiotics do. It is documented that there are fewer cases of tuberculosis in

Sandong, a province in China, where more garlic is consumed than in any other province. The antibiotic qualities of garlic can be quickly absorbed into the bloodstream by placing it directly on a cut or wound.

In India, garlic is currently being used to help dissolve blood clots in people with heart disease. Garlic does this by increasing fibrinolytic activity (the blood's ability to break down fibrin clots in the blood vessels).

American researchers have also picked up on the cardiovascular advantages of garlic. Groups who were given liberal amounts of garlic, as opposed to groups who ate none, increased their fibrinolytic activity by 130 percent in healthy people and 96 percent in people who have had recent heart attacks.

Garlic is also used for common ailments such as cold symptoms, colic in babies, coughing, chronic diarrhea, and sinus problems. Garlic has also been used to purge worms in dogs and promote general good intestinal health in all animals.

Grapes: The juice from grapes can be used as a disinfectant for cuts or abrasions of the skin. Like apples, grapes also contain boron, which could help prevent osteoporosis.

Hot peppers: Peppers may reduce the tendency of blood clotting in the arteries and stimulate mucous membranes in the respiratory tract, which helps relieve congestion.

Kiwi fruit: The kiwi contains proteolytic acid, which breaks down cholesterol in the body. It is also very rich in fiber.

Onions: This is another bulb vegetable used to treat everything from A to Z. All bulb vegetables can be used for the treatment and prevention of heart disease. They are helpful in lowering cholesterol and triglyceride levels. They also reduce the clumping of blood platelet cells that help cause the formation of plaque on the inside of the arteries, and they are a great digestive system cleanser. Onions are used in Asia as a diuretic and treatment for high blood pressure.

Papayas: This fruit contains a powerful enzyme that helps disinfect wounds and aid digestion. I recommend the concentrated form to people for gas, bloating, heartburn, and halitosis.

Pineapples: An enzyme called bromelain in the pineapple is a good digestive aid. It works in the blood vessels by reducing inflammation and keeping blood platelets from clumping. This is good news for people with coronary artery disease.

Sugar: The first time I saw sugar used medically was many years ago in a small hospital in Ohio. We used sugar on our patients who had open bedsores. The sugar remedy worked well. But it was just recently that I discovered the theory behind it: Bacteria does not grow well in sugar and the granules irritate the skin tissue to stimulate new growth and healing.

Vinegar: Vinegar has been used by many people for such things as athlete's foot, dandruff, insect bites, poison ivy, sore throat, swimmer's ear, sunburn, jellyfish stings, and toothache.

Watercress: Fresh juice from the leaves of the watercress is used to treat many kinds of skin problems, from infections to acne.

Live Juices

Fruit and vegetable juices are a wonderful way to transfer the vital life force of the plant into our bodies in a concentrated form. The nutrients and healing properties of juices are absorbed directly into the blood stream from the intestinal tract. Some examples of the juices I use for good health are:

Carrot juice: For overall good health, arthritis, and ulcers.

Beet juice: To cleanse and detoxify the liver.

Dark green vegetable juice: To provide calcium for strong bones and healthy muscles.

Cooking Smart

Preparation of food is a very important aspect of your nutrition. I would like to pass on some of my discoveries and helpful hints for preparing and serving more healthful meals. Let's start with equipment: nonstick skillets, loaf pans with drain holes, frozen dessert makers, gravy skimmers, broiler pans, woks, and vegetable steamers; these implements are designed to help you eliminate most of the fats used in cooking.

Variety Is the Spice of Life

The actual methods of cooking are also very important. They are divided into two categories: the nutrient-saving methods and the nutrient-wasting methods. The nutrient-saving methods include roasting, broiling, stewing, baking, stir frying, steaming, pressure cooking, and microwaving. The nutrient-wasting methods include charcoal broiling, frying, deep-frying, boiling, and toasting.

When you deep-fry, you add fat to the food. The intense heat involved in this process also destroys valuable nutrients—even heat-resistant vitamin A. Even though there is much controversy surrounding microwave cooking, I enjoy it. It does not heat up my kitchen during the summer months, and the quick cooking time saves on nutrients and reduces the amount of crude fat in the finished product. With a faster defrosting time, nutrients do not break down as much, and microwaved meats contain higher levels of protein because they do not brown. Browning binds the protein so it is not absorbed into the digestive tract. Use paper towels to absorb most of the fats from meats like ground beef and bacon.

A ten-year study done at Cornell University showed that vegetables cooked in one teaspoon of water retained up to 100 percent of their vitamin content. Boiling your vegetables retains only 40 to 60 percent because the soluble vitamins escape into the water. If you boil vegetables on the stove, use a very small amount of water and cook until they are just crisp. For a change, try your greens just lightly braised. They are low in calories and high in vitamins and potassium.

Cooking foods in oven-browning bags, clay pots, plastic bags, foil, parchment, and wax paper eliminates fats and retains juices. If you are roasting, do it in a pan that allows the fat to be drained during the cooking. Convection ovens, which use hot air circulation, help reduce fats and are more efficient to use than electric ovens.

Many people love the taste of grilled food. With today's new gas grills, this method of cooking has become very popular. Learn the most efficient way of using your grill so that you do not burn the food. A good method of cooking is to wrap the food in foil or place in a pan. I like to combine my meat, vegetables, and different types of soups for a one-pan, nutritious meal. The soups and all of the juices from the meats and the vegetables make the gravy.

Poaching is another method of cooking meats, fish, or poultry. I like to poach using a variety of different liquids, from vegetable juices to wine. I also try a different seasoning trick almost every time and use herbs, spices, veggies, lemons, or bulb vegetables.

Taste the Difference

There are many tricks of the trade for turning out delicious meals while cutting down on fat and salt. Cooking with alcohol is a tasty alternative to salt, and most of the alcohol evaporates in five to ten seconds. Or, you can flavor with Dijon mustard, peppers, fresh herbs, spices, and flavored vinegars. Marinating your meats before cooking enhances the flavor without salt. We all have different taste in foods, therefore, you will not know if you like something until you try it.

Check, Please

The most important factor in your diet is *you!* Take charge of your diet. Decide what food goes into your body, then decide what goes into your food. You can be a more active participant in your decisions by preparing your own food more and eating out less. More restaurants today are serving fresh food in natural ways, but they are still scarce. Eating out is a nice enjoyable treat, especially for those who do not like to cook or do not have the time, but doing your own preparation gives you more control over your food. After awhile, you may even get spoiled by preparing your own meals and not want to eat out as much.

Dress up your food. Make it look appetizing and fun to eat. Keep the process of eating interesting by using a variety of foods and combinations. You do not have to limit such things as breakfast foods to breakfast. You also do not have to eat the same things your mother used to cook. The more you try different foods, the more varied your taste will become.

Whatever you eat, savor it and enjoy it! Bless it and *know* that it will do your body some good. Eat sensibly and feed yourself a positive thought appetizer. Now that you have discovered the wonderful healing properties of the food we eat, be healthy and bon appétit!

10

Exercise

EXERCISE. THERE ARE many wonderful reasons to exercise but they usually all boil down to one primary reason—exercise is absolutely essential to your good health and well-being.

Good Excuses

For women, especially those in their latter years, vigorous exercise at least three times a week will help drive the necessary calcium back into the bones. For those with weight challenges, exercise will help increase their metabolism and burn off those extra pounds. For people with high blood pressure, exercise helps the muscles of the legs massage the long veins, helping the blood return back to the heart.

For the stressed-out population of our planet, exercise is a great release valve that will let off anxiety, frustration, and anger. In addition, exercise is an ideal time for thought and meditation.

These are but a few of the wonderful reasons for exercising. Individuals must decide for themselves the benefits they will derive from it. They must also decide where to place exercise on their priority list.

For many people, exercise is a wonderful, exhilarating experience. They enjoy the high of the adrenaline rush, which is a much better feeling than any drug because it comes with a sense of accomplishment and self-satisfaction.

Exercise Your Excuse

Other people may dread exercise and view it as a waste of expended energy. To them, it is sheer drudgery and pain. Others just don't like to sweat. As you can see, everyone's perception is truly different.

Many times you may feel too tired to exercise, especially when you are just starting. However, the more you exercise, the more energy you will have. You will find that the adrenal glands get accustomed to producing adrenaline, especially if you exercise at the same time every day. When you do not exercise, there is no reason for the extra adrenaline and energy.

Getting the Lead Out

The bottom line is: You must be painfully honest with yourself and decide if you are in need of exercise or if you need to increase the amount of exercise you are currently doing. After assessment and with the help of meditation, visualization, and affirmations, start your own exercise program. The positive mental work you do will help change your attitude toward exercise and make it physically easier for you.

Affirm every day how much you enjoy exercising and how much better it makes you feel. Visually see yourself walking vigorously with a smile and feel the energy flow through your body. This will soon become a very positive image for you and soon your attitude toward exercise may change to the point where you actually look forward to your exercise time.

The more you approach exercise with a positive attitude, and the more you concentrate on it mentally, the more you will get out of it physically. This is another step toward taking responsibility for your own health. So, enjoy it!

11

....

Healing Herbs

HEALING WITH HERBS is probably as ancient as time itself. People have been using the gifts of the earth to help heal their bodies and minds for a long time. There are written records of herbal use that date back to 5000 B.C., and many civilized cultures have used the natural healing of the earth down through the centuries.

Natural healing with herbs is still used in most of the world today. Chinese medicine relies heavily on herbal remedies with focus on prevention and strengthening the immune system. Unfortunately, most medical philosophies in our Western culture seem to fight against nature rather than work with it. Working with nature means dealing with the energies of the body to assist in natural healing.

Since ancient times, the Chinese, Egyptian, Greek, and Hindu cultures have utilized all aspects of the body, mind, and spirit to facilitate a complete and total healing of the whole person. They believe in moderation of life, diet, exercise, meditation, and being in touch with one's inner self and in tune with nature.

Plants open and aid healing forces within us.

Much of modern medicine is still based on plants. Penicillin, probably the most famous, is derived from mold that is a living organism. The rauwolfia plant extract is a component in the drug reserpine, which is used to lower blood pressure. Digitalis is made from the foxglove and has been used by many a folk healer for cardiac problems.

Herb Is Not a Guy

For many people, the use of herbs to aid healing is a natural step away from the chemicals of modern Western medicine. Even though today's medicines have their base in herbs, it seems that when the chemical structures are tampered with and made into something unnatural, it does not take long for the body to start rejecting them. This is one of the major reasons many people have turned to alternative forms of healing.

There are many of us whose physical bodies are rejecting more and more chemical preparations. I have had many reactions to the chemicals, and since I know that there are other alternatives to health, herbs became a logical choice for me.

Increasingly, the medical community has taken notice of herbs and now many researchers are starting to look into the curative power of herbs.

Various Uses of Herbs

Herbs are used in many ways to facilitate healing. They can be used to cause the body to cleanse its toxins by urinating, perspiring, defecating, sneezing, coughing, salivating, expectorating, or vomiting. Helping to stimulate the immune system is the function of the herb echinacea. Herbs can conserve or increase the body's energy. They can calm the nervous system or stimulate it. They have substances for building and nourishing the body. Many of an herb's nutrients are more concentrated and usable by the body than man-made vitamin and mineral supplements. They can stabilize organs and their systems to keep the body balanced and in good health.

A wonderful example of the traditional use of herbs is the practice of eating hot peppers by people who live in warm climates. These plants heat the body and affect the circulation by increasing the blood flow to the capillaries near the skin surface. This causes the body heat to be exposed to the skin surface where evaporation of sweat causes the body to cool off.

The Herb As a Plant

I feel the most significant contribution of a plant is the transfer of its life force energy to be used in a healing capacity. Of course, the other side of the coin is the acceptance of the energy by the person needing the healing. The plant itself does not actually do the healing. As with everything, the plant only opens and aids the marvelous healing force within us all. We must do the rest; accept the energy and the healing, and resolve whatever prompted us to manifest the disease in the first place.

You and the Herb

The use of herbs today has evolved through meditation, experimentation, and awareness of the plant and our inner selves. You too have the ability to tap into this same information and awareness. Reading books on herbs is a good way to become aware of any plants that may be harmful. The best way to learn is to get to know the herb and its properties, vibration, and effects on different parts of the body, as well as why it works. Also, listen to what your body tells you in meditation.

Our bodies know which herb is good for us and how much to take. The use of herbs is individual for each person because the herb reacts differently in each body. This is why many of the herb's reactions cannot be pinned down and documented when fed to laboratory rats.

When I recommend herbs for people, I cannot always tell them the exact amount to take. I give guidelines and advise them to "feel" their way around and let their inner awareness tell them how much to take. I have always relied on my "feelings" for such matters and have never been given false information.

The following scenario is an example of "listening to your body": I had been taking psyllium seed husks daily for bowel cleansing over a period of two to three months.

One day, as I was mixing the concoction, I felt my body say, "Enough," and right then and there I stopped taking the herb. The feeling was too strong for me to ignore.

Working with herbs needs to be done with some presence of mind. If you take too much of anything, or take it for too long, you may experience side effects or immunity to the effects of the substance. These side effects are usually the exact symptoms you are trying to treat. This is true of anything, especially chemical medicines. When I worked in a hospital, I always knew when a patient was becoming toxic on a certain drug, because they would start to exhibit the same symptoms they were being treated for. This is especially true of cardiac drugs. They seem to show the fastest and the most dramatic signs and symptoms.

In the bibliography, I have listed books I use for herbal remedies, which I highly recommend. If you are interested and wish to pursue the use of herbs, I suggest you do some reading and experimenting. Most herbs are totally benign and only aid in the healing process but, again, all of our bodies are different and the possibility of a reaction is always there. In using herbs, as with anything, *moderation* is the key word. Too much of anything can be harmful.

If you are really interested in using herbs, I suggest that you find a source for the purest grown kind or grow them yourself. This way, you are assured that no chemicals were used in the growing or processing of the herb. Here I am going to share with you some of the herbs and combinations I used and have seen successfully used by others.

Keep in mind, this is not a guidebook for herbal remedies, but an informational tool offered to make you aware of the potential benefits of plants to the human body.

Herb Stories

Alfalfa: This is a plant packed with vitamins and minerals. I have used it as a natural antihistamine. Anytime there is a problem with excess histamine, such as allergies, arthritis, ulcers, or an inflammatory problem, alfalfa can be used.

I had an acquaintance whose husband had been having cortisone injections in his shoulder for bursitis for many years. The injections only helped for a short period of time; before long the pain was back again. I suggested he take alfalfa tablets every day for at least four weeks. Before the end of the four weeks, for the first time in years, he was finally free of pain. The alfalfa worked for this man without the devastating side effects that cortisone therapy can have on the body.

There was a period in time when I accepted colds and sinus drainage. I began to take alfalfa and it seemed to clear the mucus drainage without any of the adverse reactions of chemical antihistamines.

For most of my patients with stomach or ulcer problems, I usually recommend chlorophyll or aloe juice. However, some people find that alfalfa brewed in a tea works very well for them with its antihistamine effect. After all, some of the expensive ulcer medications are mostly antihistamines.

Aloe: If any plant can work miracles, this one can. I use it for everything from cuts, burns, rashes, insect bites, sunburns, stomach upset, and ulcers to body cleansing. There is some controversy surrounding the use of aloe internally due to the fact there are little, if any, regulations on its gel extraction. I have not had any problems, nor have any of my patients, with using the aloe internally. To be on the safe side, you can do the extracting yourself and keep some bottled in the refrigerator, where it will stay fresh. I always keep aloe plants around and give them as gifts of healing love. If used in large doses, aloe may cause bowel cramping and diarrhea.

Basil: This is a wonderful herb that I use more for cooking than I do for healing. It is great for nausea and headaches and is so safe it has been used by nursing mothers to increase their milk and aid their baby's digestion. If you are pregnant or nursing, do not ingest more than the recommended daily amount of basil; do not let infants and small toddlers use internally.

Catnip: This herb has been enjoyed by cats for years, but it has many benefits for people too. I have recommended catnip to people who are trying to stop smoking; it calms their nervous system and helps them get through the initial "drying out" period. It is very beneficial when using to calm general restlessness. Catnip should not be used by pregnant women.

Chamomile: This is an ancient herb and one of the most gentle known today. One of chamomile's best uses, and the one I recommend the most, is as a sedative. It is especially good for babies who are crabby. I have prepared it as a tea and dispense it right in the bottle. It is also useful for women experiencing PMS symptoms. Some people have shown allergic reactions to chamomile, so try a very small amount first. Do not take it for prolonged periods of time. Pregnant women should consult a doctor before using chamomile.

Comfrey: This is a very powerful plant. Widely used as a poultice to heal wounds, comfrey is effective as an anti-inflammatory and can aid in burns, stings, cuts, strains, and sprains. I have also used it for my older patients as an external compress to relieve joint pain. Comfrey is not recommended for internal use while pregnant or nursing. This herb should not be used on abraded skin and should not be used on unbroken skin for prolonged periods. Recent research confirms that comfrey contains allantoin, which has been identified as an agent that stimulates new cell growth or cell proliferation. This makes it useful for wound healing, but findings indicate that certain alkaloids taken in very large quantities may be carcinogenic.

Echinacea: This is an herb I highly recommend for anyone with cold or flu symptoms, or anytime you feel your immune system needs a boost. Echinacea is a native American herb, but the Chinese have been so impressed with it, they have added it to many of their herbal combination medicines. Since it works primarily on the immune system, it is beneficial for bacterial, viral, and fungal infections. Echinacea should not be used by people who are immune-compromised.

Eyebright: This is one herb that is just as effective taken internally as externally. Externally, it has been used to soothe the irritation of inflamed eyes and promote better vision. I have also known of people who have taken it internally to increase their visual capacity.

Fenugreek: This herb has many uses, from soothing the bowel to promoting breast milk production. I have used the seeds brewed as a tea for chest congestion. Fenugreek can be used as a poultice on boils and sores to draw out waste. Do not ingest the seeds if you are pregnant.

Feverfew: This herb has been used by several medical doctors for the treatment of migraine headaches and was even discussed in one of the more prominent medical journals. Feverfew's anti-inflammatory actions are also great for arthritis. Do not ingest if you are pregnant or nursing.

Garlic: This is probably one of the most versatile and ancient healing plants on the earth. Its antibiotic qualities can be used for virtually every part of the body. In Asia and many parts of Europe, garlic is used as treatment for high blood pressure. Many people in the United States have found that garlic does a much better job in controlling their blood pressure without the side effects of conventional drugs. Garlic is not recommended for those with inflammatory conditions, fevers, and thin blood. Garlic capsules and extract should not be used during pregnancy or while nursing.

Ginger: This is another extremely versatile herb. Ginger originated in China where it has been widely used by commoners, nonprofessionals, and professional healers alike. It is used for colds and flu-like symptoms because it is helpful in the elimination of mucus production. Ginger is said to warm and strengthen the vital organs, and has been used for hangovers and overall body weakness. Compresses are used to relieve body aches, pains, arthritis, and menstrual cramps. A foot bath and massage with ginger oil is said to promote better circulation in the body. It can also be used to ease indigestion and gas in the lower bowel. Ginger capsules are not to be used during pregnancy. Persons with gallstones should consult a health care practitioner before using capsules.

Ginseng: This herb has been reputed to have an illumination all its own and to move around at night. Ginseng has many wonderful healing properties. The Chinese have used it for years to strengthen the body's endurance and increase resistance to infection. It contains substances similar to the female hormone estrogen; therefore, it offers a more natural way to deal with estrogen imbalance caused by menopause. Ginseng has also been used for senility, diabetes, anemia, stomach problems, and headaches. Ginsing has been known to raise blood pressure. If you have hypertension, consult your physician. Pregnant women should use ginsing with caution.

Goldenseal root: This herb has traditional antibiotic and antiseptic effects. I once knew a lady who used it to save her dog's life after the veterinarian had given up. Goldenseal can be taken internally as a tea, or used externally as a powder sprinkled directly on a wound. Use of goldenseal root can cause hypertension. It should be used with caution. Long-term use is not recommended. Pregnant or nursing women should not use goldenseal.

Horehound: I remember as a child my mother giving me horehound cough drops for my colds. At the time, I wasn't aware that they were an old herbal preparation; I just knew they worked. Other uses for horehound are to break fevers, serve as a laxative, soothe itches and rashes, and expel worms. Do not ingest while pregnant.

Horseradish: I have used this herb and have recommended it for years for clearing the sinuses. Other uses have been to ease chest congestion and muscle aches and pains. As with many of the herbs, do not exceed the normal food levels. Children under the age of four may have trouble digesting horseradish. If you have kidney disorders or gastric inflammation, you should not ingest horseradish unless approved by your doctor.

Ipecacuanha: This herb is commonly known as ipecac and is used in hospital emergency rooms and homes as an agent to induce vomiting for internal poisoning. Do not use this herb in large quantities, as it may cause uncontrolled vomiting and gastric distress.

Parsley: One of the most nutritious herbs, parsley is packed with vitamins A and C, calcium, thiamin, riboflavin, and niacin. As I have explained elsewhere, parsley is excellent for detoxifying the liver and bloodstream in general. Europeans use it as a mouth freshener after their meals. It can also be used as a laxative or diuretic; therefore, if you have kidney problems, avoid large quantities. Pregnant women should not use more than recommended amount due to its effect on the kidneys and liver.

Pennyroyal: This herb is one of the best-smelling insect repellents I know of. I use the oil mixed with baby shampoo as flea soap for my cats. You can also crush the fresh leaves on your body for a good insect repellent of your own. Ingesting pennyroyal is not recommended, especially while nursing or pregnant. Internal use may cause diarrhea and harm the kidneys and liver. I recommend that you only use it externally as an insect repellent.

Raspberry leaf: Before I learned relaxation and visualization techniques, I used this tea to help relieve my menstrual cramps. For years, both Chinese and European women have taken it during pregnancy to prepare themselves for childbirth.

Uva ursi: This herb is also called bearberry. I am grateful to this herb for getting me off the antibiotic merry-go-round. It is safe to use for long-term urinary problems and will not interfere with your immune system. I usually take it as an extract, but for fast relief of a painful bladder infection, the whole leaves can be chewed. If you have severe kidney problems, you should not use this herb. Large doses or long-term use can cause upset stomach and digestive and gastrointestinal irritation. Pregnant women should not use Uva ursi.

Valerian: This herb works great not only as a muscle relaxant but also as a nervous system relaxant. I have safely given it to adults, children, babies, and cats. If I find myself baby sitting, I make sure I have plenty of valerian on hand! Very young children do not respond predictably to valerian. Refrain from using it on infants and toddlers.

God's Gifts in Many Forms

This is just a very small sampling of herbs available and their actions. Some can be combined for different results; some are to be used alone. They can be used as teas, poultices, soaks, oils for infusion, oils for massage, baths, salves, ointments, liniments, compresses, syrups, lotions, suppositories, and powders. Nature's healing garden is virtually unlimited in its gifts.

Many foods with herbs are also included in this wonderful repertoire and they are covered in the food section.

Herbs are a great way to get back in touch with nature and become balanced. They are some of God's wonderful gifts to mankind to be used with love and respect. If you are game, you too can open up a wonderful world of love through plants.

As a health-care professional, I see many people who are not well served by modern medical prescriptions and treatments. The use of herbal remedies can be a welcome and successful change that encourages personal power and will lead to a healthier way of life.

Like any product, natural or synthetic, there are some precautions to heed with herbal alternatives. Most cautions involve pregnant and lactating women. Some herbs can be harmful if taken in large doses or over extended periods of time. Likewise, combining herbal products with prescription drugs can alter their effectiveness.

As you review the herbs I have discussed, keep in mind that these act as drugs in the system and should be used with caution and not without full knowledge of all ingredients and possible side effects.

12

··

The Power of Touch

THERE IS ONE type of alternative healing that may be familiar to many of you, but in different forms. It is called hands-on healing. Some have seen it done in religious settings, others have been exposed to it in folklore, and some have read about it in magazines or seen it on television. Whatever your method of exposure, hands-on healing is a very interesting and helpful experience.

The Human Touch

The touch of the human hand brings forth many varied perceptions and feelings. For some who have had negative experiences from being touched, it can be uncomfortable. These people need to do much inner healing and resolution to reap the benefits of positive touch. For most of us, human touch is positive and reassuring. This feeling starts at birth with the physical, mental, and emotional bonding of a baby to its parent.

Some of the many studies that have been conducted on human touch reveal that touch can increase hemoglobin (the part of the blood that carries oxygen) in the body. The immune system can also be stimulated by the loving, compassionate approach of the person applying the therapy. Touch can help relieve pain through the release of endorphins, which are morphine-like substances produced by our bodies.

Other physical effects of touch on the body are the assistance of venous and lymphatic flow throughout the body and stretching of the muscles. Touch is very beneficial for stress reduction and promoting relaxation, and it aids in the removal of toxins in the body.

There have been many studies done that demonstrate the harmful effects that touch depravation can have on babies and children. Many totally shut down and withdraw into themselves, excluding any real contact with the outside world. So, without question, touch is very important to human growth and development at any age.

My Technique

My preferred method of doing therapeutic touch has evolved over a period of time with continued learning and growth. This technique works best for me now; however, tomorrow I might chance upon something new and integrate that into the healing process as well.

The first thing I do in a therapeutic touch session is focus myself by visually centering on my chakras. Next, I visualize the top of my head open with white light energy coming into it from the universe and flowing throughout my body and finally coming out of my hands. I then tune into the person's energy to establish a telepathic connection and I very lightly run my hands about an inch above the surface of their skin in the affected area. I usually can feel heat or a tingling of some kind. Next, I start making wiping motions with my hand to brush away the pain vibration coming from the area.

The next step is to get the person involved. I tell them to release the pain and let it go. I ask them to picture the pain flowing out of their body and into the ground.

Useful Examples

Of course, depending on the circumstances of the pain, there can be a lot more involved with the releasing of pain or disease. I will give you two examples:

I was once working with a lady, balancing her body energy and doing a general body healing, when I picked up a sharp pain in her stomach. I asked her if she was aware of it and she confirmed she was. I then asked her to visualize the area filled with soothing pink light and mentally release the pain. After the session, we both realized she needed to work on many issues in her life that needed healing. These issues were "eating at her" and she was manifesting it in her solar plexus area. This behavior is frequently the cause of ulcers.

Another person I worked on was more open and willing to explore the source of his pain immediately. He was having terrific muscle spasms in his back, and the pain was so intense that he needed a cane to stand upright enough to walk. As I brushed away the pain energy field, we talked about when and why the pain started. He told me he was bent over his computer trying to type a bill for some equipment that had been taken from him. He was doing this with much anger and resentment. He agreed that he should just let the incident go and with it, his anger and resentment. I started doing some pressure massage and could feel the muscles loosening and becoming soft and pliable under my fingers. He felt much better and agreed to go home and work on releasing the whole incident.

More than One Way

Even though I have always had the ability to work with telepathic healing, my interest was aroused a few years ago when I read a book on therapeutic touch written by Dolores Krieger. Her technique, which involves smoothing out an unbalanced energy field and balancing the body, is simple and is now being taught in many nursing schools around the country. In part of her teachings is the concept of the need for human compassion and caring, which enables us to help others. As a result, nurses are becoming more aware of the impact their touch has on their patients. Today, many nurses are incorporating touch with their desire to have a positive healing impact on the people they care for.

Touch therapies that are more involved include therapeutic massage and acupressure. A therapist who spends time taking courses in anatomy and physiology and therapeutic touch usually does both. Some schools require as much as 1,200 hours of textbook and practical instruction for certification or graduation. Some of their studies may include the following methods of touch:

Kinesiology and palpation: The study of muscles and how they work.

Effleurage: A stroking that glides over the skin with firm and even pressure. This method of touch is used to find areas of soreness or tightness or to provide a passive, stretching motion to the muscles.

Petrissage: A kneading motion of the muscles to help "milk" the muscles of any tissue or cellular waste that accumulates in a muscle that is not frequently used.

Acupressure: A therapy that involves using pressure with a thumb, hand, or elbow over a pressure point on the body. These points usually correspond to acupuncture points. The points are designed to stimulate certain healing activities in the body, including the relief of pain.

Polarity: The technique of working with and balancing energies that flow through the body.

To give professional credibility to the massage therapist and ensure quality therapy, most states now require licensing of all massage therapists. National certification will soon be required too.

Asking "Why?"

Again, most of what healing is about is, "Why did I manifest this in the first place?" Consciously or subconsciously, and for whatever reason, we do it to ourselves. Of course, it takes blunt honesty and sometimes deep soul searching to find out why. Remember also that as you grow and evolve, your perceptions of life change. If you manifested a sore back for one reason as a young adult, that same manifestation may be for a different reason later in life.

Remember to Love

Always remember, whenever you are working with anyone using touch, use it with love and compassion. Do not concern yourself with the "whys" of the other person's manifestation or judge them in any way. This only interferes with your transfer of healing energy. You are using negative energy by judging someone else's actions, thus inhibiting the flow of the pure white-light healing energy that you are capable of channeling.

13

....

The Aging Process

I AM ALWAYS on the lookout for ideas to enrich my life and writing. One night I was watching television and tuned into a PBS special that made me really stop and think about the aging process. As a society, it is amazing to me how caught up we are in the evolution of getting older. We appear to be a youth-oriented culture. Personally, I don't have a problem with the natural process of maturing. To me, aging is as much a part of our lives and experiences on this earth plane as being born and growing up.

No one should fear living from age thirty to age eighty any more than living from age one to thirty. Buying into the fear of aging will do nothing but make it worse. Fear of anything gives it strength. If we have a morbid fear of getting mugged in the park, more than likely we will draw that experience to us; but, if we know the universe protects us and feel it in our hearts and whole being, we have nothing to fear.

Training Wheels

You would think there would be more apprehension in the transition from age one to thirty. For instance, look at all of the body changes we go through. If pressed, we usually can't recognize a twenty-year-old from his baby picture, and mental and emotional changes are even more powerful than physical changes. Growing up is not the easiest thing we will do in our lives, but I don't see any five-year-old searching the Yellow Pages for a spa to stave off puberty.

On the contrary, most children can't wait to "grow up" and become adults. In fact, these days children are pushing it at a faster rate than ever before. Ironically, when we are young, we want to be older, and when we are old, we want to be young again. I think it's time we make up our minds.

Aging Is a Gray Area

For some reason, society tells us that the teen years to forty is the only place to be. If we are older than forty, we are over the hill—*aging*. This is where fear develops. Most people see aging as the beginning of illness, senility, helplessness, and loneliness. Unfortunately, this is the image that is portrayed in the media and is what some people have created for themselves.

It does not have to be that way.

There are many people who are thoroughly enjoying their retirement or have chosen not to retire at all. For some, this is the most creative, fulfilling time of their lives. Later years are when most of the obligations and responsibilities of life have been lifted and people can follow the dreams they have held on to for so long. Again—

The world we live in is what we have created.

My father and a friend of his are both in their seventies but you would never know it if you looked at them. They have the appearance of being in their fifties and the attitude of people in their thirties. They have not adopted the "I'm just going to sit down and wait to die" mindset. If they did, that is exactly what would happen. Of course, I have also met people in their thirties with this resigned attitude, so retirees do not have the corner on this market.

You Are My Sunshine

Living in southern Florida, I am constantly exposed to older people and have found they come in all varieties. The ones with the best attitudes are certainly the happiest and healthiest. They are the ones who have discovered how to turn lemons into lemonade. Most have moved to the Sunshine State for a specific reason and when there is no sunshine, they create their own.

They have learned many wonderful lessons as they journey down the path of life and use them to their fullest extent. These are also the people whose ages can't be guessed. Most have not gotten caught up in the "aging syndrome." They do not feed into their maturity one of our most powerful emotions—*fear*. Someday, people will realize—

Fearing something gives it power to materialize.

On the other side of the coin are those who want to age. They use the process of aging as some use illness; they use it as an excuse and form of control to manipulate others, especially their own family members and friends. Control over others is just an illusion, and a dubious one at that.

We must honestly look at ourselves and see
how we manifest our reality.

An Ounce of Prevention

Prevention is the name of the health game any time. This is especially true with a maturing body; for prevention is one of the best ways to grow older gracefully. Taking care of ourselves as we live our lives one day at a time is an ideal way of preventing many aging problems.

A Taste-Budding Experience

A good balanced diet with a minimum of processed foods and alcohol, a lot of raw fruits, vegetables, and fiber, and plenty of fluids takes care of what goes into our body. A diet rich in vitamins and minerals is a bonus to all parts of the body, including the brain.

Tasting good food is one of our more enjoyable pastimes. However, there are many older people who cannot appreciate the taste of any food. These people lose interest in eating and begin a downward spiral of malnutrition. The good news is that zinc is the nutritional supplement that can perk up the taste buds and provide a new outlook on life, or at least what we eat. Without zinc, the taste buds cannot differentiate between tastes. Everything seems to be tasteless, thus unappetizing. Zinc is essential to the older body in other ways. Diabetics who increase their zinc and chromium intake may require less insulin. Also, zinc supplements have saved many men from unnecessary prostate surgery.

How, when, and where you eat is also very important. Eating at any age should not be stressful. It should take place at a relaxed enjoyable time of the day. We intuitively know which eating patterns work best for us and what we enjoy the most.

Clean Up

Attention to good hygiene is just as important to health as eating and is a must for everyone. Some sunshine, soap and water and, if you desire, a light coat of makeup will do more for your facial expression than all the expensive creams and injections in the world. Smoking causes wrinkles, so if you are smoking and this is a worry, stop. Your body will love you for it. Dress sensibly and comfortably for all kinds of weather. Dressing in younger, classic styles often helps older people feel and look younger, so be open to trying new fashions.

A Breath of Fresh Air

Regular exercise, even if it is walking three times a week, is great for all parts of the body. You can exercise by yourself for quality alone time, or participate with others for group sports and activities. Both methods are very beneficial to your well-being. A good workout three times a week is essential for driving calcium back into the bones where it belongs. Without question, keeping active is one of the surest ways of staving off the "old age" syndrome.

Speaking of calcium, antacids are another hitch in the calcium story because they cause the body to secrete phosphorus from the bones. If you need something to settle your stomach, I recommend that you chew on some papaya enzyme.

Keep Busy

To stay active, do something for yourself or take an interest in an activity. Read, take up hobbies, be creative, or take classes at the local college or public schools. Get more involved with your family and community.

One behavior I can never understand is when a group of older people get together to talk about each other's medical problems. If this much power and energy is given to a problem, it is sure to overwhelm the afflicted person.

Today, I see so many older people barricading themselves in their homes. They appear to have nothing better to do than watch everyone around them and spend the rest of the time complaining about what they have seen. There is absolutely no reason for this behavior—get out and do something! For instance, there are usually golf courses around condominium complexes. If you are not a golfer, go out and walk on designated pathways or visit a park or beach. See how much goodwill you can spread to the people around you.

Age Like Wine

There is also a self-worthiness issue to consider with regard to the aging process. Again, I think the more we love ourselves, the more we are taking care of our body and mind, no matter what our age. Doctors say that when we age, our immune system decreases, leading to countless medical problems. Loving ourselves can ward off potential complications.

Some people feel that because they are older, they are no longer first-class citizens. Here we are dealing with the issue of self-worthiness again. Lack of self-worth will shut the body systems down and one of the first to go is the immune system. Look at all the happy, healthy seniors around and you will begin to realize that happiness and a healthy body, positive attitude, and great self-esteem go hand-in-hand. We should always have a positive, loving attitude—no matter what age we are. Being judgmental and resentful of others, especially young people, is a one-way street to the "old age home." Those feelings and emotions will stiffen anyone faster than super glue, for they stifle any free-flowing love felt for ourselves or anyone else. Many times we see things in people we don't like; however, much of this is behavior we have already worked through ourselves and we don't like to be reminded of it. We need to recognize this fact, be proud that we have grown in wisdom and thought, and allow others the space to work out their lessons in their own time.

More than Pets

Animals are often an overlooked source of love and goodwill. I have seen older people who were thought to be hopeless make a beautiful comeback when something soft and furry or feathery came into their lives. An animal is a being who will love you unconditionally and whom you can love in return.

Pets can also provide a purpose in life; it is human nature to rally to the cause when we feel we are needed. Unfortunately, I see many places for rent in Florida that ban pets. The reasons for such a ban are many, but the majority of places feel pets are a bother and nuisance. A well-cared-for pet is a nuisance only to those who wish to make it so.

Not allowing senior citizens who live alone to have a pet only makes their situation worse. Pets have the innate ability to ignite the spark of love and companionship in one who is lonely; and yes, the old adage is true, "The more love you give, the more you get in return."

Snooze, You Lose

I refuse to hear the excuse that an older person cannot learn something new just because they are old. The brain does not start deteriorating just because of age, but it will slow down from lack of use.

What is not used is lost.

Our memory is only as good as we want it to be. I knew a lady in her nineties who could tell you the name of every president of the United States and the order in which they served. She could also recite almost every poem she had written in her entire life, which were many. She was a loving, warm human being with many friends and she always had a kind word for everyone she met. She refused to buy into the concept of mind deterioration.

Today, there are many books written specifically about mental gymnastics. Pick up a couple, work with them, and try some of the suggestions on your kids or grand-kids. Senility seems to be a big fear (there's that word again) based on the myth that brain cells die as we age. The brain has an infinite number of possibilities for functioning. Try working with some of the 87 percent they say we never use.

Many times senility is due to nothing more than a nutritional deficiency, drugs, depression, or a small stroke. All of these possibilities should be checked out before anyone moves into the "old folks home."

Heaven Will Wait

I disagree with the way the media and medical associations set up negative thinking about aging. They usually begin sentences with, "Now that you are older and everything is falling apart." For me, this conjures visions of an arm falling off or a gall bladder dropping to the floor with a resounding splat. I don't let anyone put those thoughts in my head. People only fall apart as much as they want to. How much of this type of thinking has been programmed in us already? It doesn't matter. Don't accept it. Start reprogramming today!

Working in hospitals in southern Florida for a number of years has given me a chance to talk to hundreds of older people. The ones who had the fewest medical problems had basically the same attitude—positive. They feel that life is a challenge and that there are still many things to do out there. They don't have time to sit around and rehash any of the problems of their lives. In fact, most don't even consider having problems, just challenges and learning experiences. They adopt the same attitude toward the passing years as they do toward every other aspect of their lives, and they are committed to getting every drop of happiness out of every day they live.

Buying into Dying

Another fear that runs rampant in our older society is the fear of dying. No matter what beliefs a person may have about life after death, it is a reality we all must face eventually. I have one thought on the subject:

Instead of hanging onto the fear of dying, enjoy life.

Remember that thoughts are things and if we keep creating certain scenarios in our minds, we will soon create them in our three-dimensional reality. Visualize wonderful things happening for you. See this as the beautiful world it is and, above all, have the concept of self-love. Love of ourselves is most important.

A Good Book

There are many good books on the market today written about the aging process. One of the best I have read is the one written through collaboration with *Prevention Magazine*. It is called *Aging Slowly*. The book contains a lot of great information for healthy living at any age.

Only we can change things in our lives.

Only we can take the responsibility to have a healthy positive life. Don't depend on someone else to do it for you. Others have their own responsibilities and path to follow. We create our own reality. If we decide to go to an expensive spa in Europe to have sheep parts injected into our body to make us feel younger, that is what we will get.

Whatever we believe will become reality.

If we believe that adopting a loving, positive attitude will bring us the feeling of youth beyond our dreams, that will be our reality.

That is what being human is all about, and why we are here—to learn all we can and use the knowledge for our personal growth.

14

....

Animals and Their Health

MANY OF THE same healing techniques used for people will work for animals. They are such loving creatures, naturally do not have self-worth problems, and are capable of loving people unconditionally. This makes their acceptance of love and healing from others very easy. To share from your heart with them is not a problem.

Learn from the Animals

It is unfortunate that many people do not spend more time learning from animals. If something is wrong in your life or you are ill, animals instinctively know and are there to comfort you and share their love. People need to be open and receptive to receive the tremendous amount of love and sharing from animals.

There are many lessons we can learn from animals, especially those of humility and enjoying the simple pleasures of life. Animals are completely in tune with nature and the wonders of the earth; they can teach us how to

175

keep our lives simple and uncluttered and how to relax and put our priorities in place; they can teach us patience and how to play (something that too many of us forget how to do). Tuning into our animals is like exploring a completely different world.

Animals have many admirable qualities. Besides the ability to love unconditionally, they are honest and straightforward. They are very brave when need be. More than once, I have seen a mother cat make hamburger out of the nose of a dog many times her size while protecting her kittens. Animals are very devoted parents, many times adopting others who are not of their own species. I once had a cat that adopted a bird.

Talk to the Animals

Communication with animals is very important. I never stop talking to mine. Sometimes I even call them to dinner telepathically and it works. If you take a cat from Texas and put him with a cat from China, they will be able to communicate very well. Unfortunately, humans have difficulty communicating with each other even when they speak the same language!

Animals are very intelligent creatures. For the most part, they respond to the manner in which we treat them. If we treat them as ignorant beings without any reasoning ability, they may act as such; conversely, if we speak to them and explain things to them, we get a totally different reaction. I always explain things to my cats, especially when taking them to the veterinarian. Given an explanation of what a "shot" is, for example, makes a great deal of difference in an animal's behavior. The result is a much more cooperative animal.

A Pet for Life

For most people who live alone, an animal is a wonderful source of company for all of the above reasons. For many, their pets are the main reason for continuing to live. Where families and human companions may pass them over for other activities, their animals are faithfully there.

For people with illnesses such as stroke, paralysis, Alzheimer's disease, mental disorders, or any other major debilitating problems, animals have been known to be one of the few sources of contact. I have seen some of these people respond to the soft love of an animal when all other human attempts to reach them have failed.

Animal Health

One of the best ways to keep an animal healthy is the same way to keep us healthy—prevention. A healthy diet, exercise, clean surroundings, positive thought, and a lot of love work wonders for any pet. I feed my cats natural food without any preservatives. Sometimes I even make a turkey and vegetable stew with brown rice that I put through the food processor for them. This takes a little extra time, but I enjoy doing it and know exactly what is going into their food. Another advantage is, ounce for ounce, homemade meals can be cheaper than commercial cat food.

I have done a lot of reading on animal nutrition and I do some vitamin supplementation. Please don't do this without doing some research first. An animal's system is geared for a natural diet in the wild and a deficiency of something vital could result in a sick animal. Listed in the bibliography are several books that I used for guidelines.

Along with good nutrition, I recommend yearly checkups with a good veterinarian; one who is willing to go along with the natural approach and not fight you every step of the way. I also believe very strongly in vaccines for prevention. I use homeopathic and herbal remedies for my cats instead of traditional medicines. For example, adding vitamin C to the diet of neutered male cats may help deter bladder problems that can plague them. Acidophilus for diarrhea is natural and much more sensible than something that interferes with the natural body functions. In addition, it works without upsetting the delicate balance of the animal's system.

Exercise is another important factor in an animal's health. Make sure ample exercise is provided for your pet, whether it is going for walks, letting him run in an enclosed yard, or playing in the house. I have contrived several games with my cats, including tag. We play it outside and inside.

Don't Eat the Daisies

Cats, dogs, and birds love to chew on plants. This can be dangerous for your pets, especially if they chew on a plant that is harmful to them. Some plants have deadly poisons in their leaves, seeds, berries, or flowers that can affect the animals nervous, gastrointestinal, or cardiovascular systems, and may even cause death. There are many different signs and symptoms that an animal can exhibit when in distress. Be aware of any abnormal behavior in your pets: excessive salivation, labored breathing, skin rashes, or bloody urine. Contact your veterinarian if you suspect your pet has eaten something poisonous. Examples of poisonous plants are azalea, dieffenbachia, elephant ears, ivy (all varieties), philodendron, poinsettia, and rhododendron.

No Bones About It

Animals are probably the most receptive creatures to healing. They have no preconceived notions of health. Animals hold themselves in very high esteem; therefore, they do not have feelings of guilt and are very open to accepting love. They are not programmed for illness by the Western medical philosophy.

Because animals do not watch television, they are not exposed to the advertising focused on stomach indigestion, headaches, allergies, and the like, so they are not normally bothered by these ailments unless they eat or do something totally unnatural to themselves. They have an unlimited amount of patience and are not looking for the "fast, fast relief" that an artificial chemical can give.

Animals also seem to know what is best for them and they do it—they eat grass for an upset stomach caused by eating too many lizards, or they sleep a lot and let the body rest for many of their minor ailments.

Animals do not use illness for secondary gains; for example, extra attention. However, animals are very smart and many will pick up on the fact that being sick can have its advantages at times. Giving animals a lot of positive reinforcement and love when they are healthy will show them that they will get love whether they are ill or well.

Healing Touch

As I have talked before about the power of human touch and the intent to heal, the same applies for animals. Dr. Michael Fox has written a great book on animal massage called *The Healing Touch*. He has wonderful insight into the power of natural healing and the book is a must for anyone who loves animals. Animals really love healing, especially hands-on. They know that it comes from our hearts to their hearts. They have the capacity for feeling pure love and accepting it totally. That is only one important lesson we can learn from them.

The Fur Ball

I have done healing two different ways on my animals. About two years ago, my female cat had a large fur ball stuck in her stomach. She became very sick, and I thought I might lose her. For three days I force-fed her vitamins, mineral oil, and fluids. She just kept getting worse. On the third night, I went into meditation and mentally made contact with her.

I visually saw the fur ball in her stomach, pulled it out mentally with my fingers, and disposed of it. I then soothed the area with green light and surrounded her with a nourishing, healing white light. The next morning, she was her old self, eating everything in sight. She was very happy and content and I knew she was fine. Again, remember that I am a health-care professional and experienced healer. If you are uncertain of the symptoms or treatment, seek the advice of a veterinarian.

Fleas Be Gone

Another story involves the time my male cat received an overdose of flea spray. I usually use only natural remedies on my cats, but the fleas were getting the best of us and the situation was becoming desperate. The chemicals made him very sick. He sat hunched on the bed with his eyes dilated and his mouth drooling. I put my hands around his body and could feel how sick he was. He was very nauseated and had a horrible pain in his stomach.

I covered us both with white healing light while I breathed in fresh air and breathed out the pain. Within seconds, he was fine and got up purring and ready to play again. I had taken his pain into my body and gotten rid of it for both of us. I do not suggest doing this unless you are very confident in your ability to release the pain and get rid of it yourself. This is not something I do very often, but I knew the method would work quickly.

Paws-On Healing

I had another incident with my male cat that I'd like to share with you. One night he crawled into the house with an injured rear leg. It looked as though he had fallen out of a tree and caught his foot in the branches. The foot itself was scraped and bleeding. It was hot to the touch and swollen. His upper leg was very swollen and he could not be touched without squealing in pain. I called the veterinarian and was told he could not see him until the next morning.

I knew I had to do something for him before morning. His body was hot, his pupils dilated, and he continued to scream in pain. The calming pink light didn't seem to work. (This was probably because I was so emotionally involved and was having a hard time settling myself down). I had some valerian root tea that I brewed for him, and with a medicine dropper, I was able to get it down. I put him in a dark confined space and left him alone.

I then centered myself, went into a deep meditation, and mentally contacted him. I could see in my mind's eye that he had no broken bones, just a lot of torn ligaments and tendons. The muscles were swollen and inflamed. In my mind, I immediately wrapped all of the bones with green healing light (just in case I had missed something). Next, I covered all of the muscles and nerves with an ice-blue light to soothe and relieve the pain, and I wrapped him completely in white light. About two to three minutes into this meditation, he stopped screaming and became very quiet. I did not hear a sound from him the entire night.

The next morning my cat was much better. He could bear weight on his injured leg without much pain. The heat and swelling had gone down and the cuts had scabbed over and were almost healed. I took him to our veterinarian for a good checkup. The veterinarian was able to move the foot and leg around and feel the bones without causing any discomfort. He said there was no reason to X-ray him, since there was no evidence of any major trauma. The cat continued to improve and by the end of the day his cuts were almost totally healed and the fur was starting to grow back.

All God's Creatures

Clearly, many of the same principles of caring for animals apply to caring for ourselves. We are all wonderful creatures of this earth plane and are here together for a reason. When we accept the fact that we all share the same space and when we allow each other just to be, we will have truly evolved into a higher realm of love and understanding. Animals can help us attain that understanding.

If we believe that adopting a loving, positive attitude will bring us the feeling of youth beyond our dreams, that will be reality.

15

....

Living with AIDS

WHEN I ORIGINALLY started this project, I knew very little about AIDS or the people who had the disease. Since then, I have worked with several AIDS clients and have gained insight into the illness and the many reasons people manifest the disease. As of this writing, I live in southwest Florida, in a county that ranks third in the nation for increases in reported cases of HIV infection. It is now a well-known fact that AIDS affects people of all income brackets, age levels, and social status.

Fear

There is a tremendous amount of negative energy generated by the media regarding AIDS, which has inspired large waves of fear in the general population about the disease.

This public fear about AIDS has touched and continues to touch many people who do not understand the disease or the transmission of it. Thankfully, many of those affected by AIDS, as well as their families and friends, are putting a lot of effort into public education.

There are still people who want to condemn and pass judgment on those afflicted with AIDS, but I feel there are many more open-minded, understanding, and loving people emerging and changing their viewpoint about the disease.

Recipe for Life

My approach to counseling AIDS patients is based on achieving and maintaining balance and harmony of the body, mind, and spirit. During the course of treatments, we use nutritional therapy that includes natural juicing with fresh fruits and vegetables. Emphasis is placed on carrot and beet juice for cellular rebuilding and toxin cleansing. Many of the medications taken by AIDS patients are extremely toxic to the body and accumulate in the liver. Beet juice is wonderful for helping the liver rid itself of the toxic byproducts of medication.

Herbs also play an important role in the natural healing process. Echinacea is essential for boosting the immune system, while goldenseal and garlic, both natural antibiotics, help to protect against the opportunistic infections that seem to plague many people with AIDS. Many other herbs and herbal combinations can be used as each individual situation arises.

I use meditation, guided imagery, and color therapy for physical healing. During the guided meditations, I have clients visualize the old, damaged cells removed from their bodies, put into a garbage bag, and thrown away. We then go on to rebuild new cells and cellular structures. The color green is used to wrap and coat the new cells and protect them from further damage. Pink is often used to soothe irritated areas of the body; for example, the intestinal tract or inflamed lungs.

My clients and I usually wind things up with a powerful white light pulsating in the area of the thymus gland. This light spreads throughout the body and remains with the person. This type of guided imagery works well in a meditative state. I also suggest that the person review the visualization many times during the day as one would verbal affirmations.

Emotional and spiritual healing can be accomplished through affirmations and building on a strong belief system. The affirmations are a wonderful way to rebuild self-esteem and self-love.

Endless Possibilities

I did not start out to cure anyone of AIDS, but to enhance and prolong the quality of lives. What I have witnessed is an incredible change in these people and their lives. I have seen much of their lab work show marked improvements and, in many instances, return to normal values and stay there. In addition, some have had rises in their white blood cell counts that have enabled them to discontinue specific medications.

I no longer call my clients AIDS patients, but AIDS survivors, or people living with HIV. I would now like to relate to you the story of one such survivor who plans on living past the ripe old age of ninety-two, and I have absolutely no doubt he will do it!

Daniel's Story

Daniel is a client of mine who was diagnosed with AIDS several years ago. I first met him in the hospital where he was recovering from a bout of PCP (pneumocystic carinii pneumonia). Over a short period of time, Daniel has learned the importance of having empathy for those who display ignorance toward AIDS, found the courage to come forward publicly and acknowledge his disease, and gained enormous strength and personal power in taking charge of his physical, mental, and spiritual health.

Prior to discovering he had contracted the disease, Daniel was an avid party person who occasionally abused alcohol and drugs. At the time, he thought he was happy, but looking back he knows he ignored the warning signs telling him to change his precarious lifestyle. Unfortunately for Daniel, as with many others, it took AIDS to stop him.

Daniel does not look at AIDS as a death sentence, but as a new way of life. His transition to the enthusiastic and alive person he is today was not easy. Daniel has worked many long hours to establish his priorities, realize the meaning of life, and rid himself of needless guilt and negative feelings about himself. He finally feels he is deserving of love and acceptance—a new concept he is beginning to feel comfortable with.

Daniel works tirelessly to establish a quality life for himself and maintain a close relationship with his family and friends—his primary support system. He is very regimented in maintaining his healthy lifestyle; he meditates at least twice a day, juices daily, and his affirmations and visualizations are repeated so many times that he finds them happening unconsciously. In his spare time, Daniel volunteers his services to help other HIV patients.

Loving Band-Aids

Daniel and I spend about two hours per session, once or twice a week, discussing the many aspects and implications of AIDS and the effect it has on his life. We also use positive affirmations as part of Daniel's new lifestyle and healing process. Some of the affirmations change as he progresses through his healing. Since his affirmations are all spoken in the present tense, Daniel has been able to bring the future of his good health into his present reality.

At the end of each session, Daniel and I do a meditation together in which I take him through a guided-imagery journey. We both do the visualization and work on the parts of his body that need attention. In this relaxed and focused state, Daniel is able to mentally remove the diseased portions of his body, such as the parts of his lungs damaged by the pneumonia, and throw them away in little garbage bags.

We then start the most important process—the rebuilding of new tissue. This is done cell by cell, to include the blood vessels surrounding the cellular structure. The new area of his lungs now functions perfectly and is resistant to disease. The last thing we do before the meditation is complete is to affirm the disease is over and that his experience with AIDS is complete. Of course, the sessions always end with a loving bear hug and very warm feelings.

Personal Power

Within one month of beginning sessions with Daniel, he was able to stop taking the medication that increased his white blood cell count. Today, during the guided imagery part of his meditation, Daniel pictures himself as a healthy young man giving to others the power of health and love of self—something he has gained.

Even though the numbers on Daniel's lab work look good, the best part about his story is that he *feels great!* Daniel is now out in the community, working with other PLWAs (people living with AIDS), and visiting the hospital to bring enthusiasm and positive thought to those in confinement. He speaks to various groups in the area about how he is successfully living with HIV, and is planning on going back to work soon. Daniel has done more

for himself than lie in bed, take drugs, and wait for someone to cure him—much more.

*Like Daniel, each of you has the ability to be
living testament to the healing power of the
body, mind, and spirit.*

Bibliography

Anderson, David, M.D., Dale Buegel, M.D., and Dennis Chernin, M.D. *Homeopathic Remedies for Physicians, Laymen and Therapists.*

Ballentine, Roudolph, M.D. *Diet and Nutrition—A Holistic Approach.* Honesdale, Pennsylvania: Himalayan International Institute of Yoga Science and Philosophy, 1978.

Bibb, Benjamin O. and Joseph J. Weed. *Amazing Secrets of Psychic Healing.* West Nyack, New York: Parker Publishing Co. Inc., 1976.

Bricklin, Mark, et al. *Rodale's Encyclopedia of Natural Home Remedies.* Emmaus, Pennsylvania: Rodale Press Inc., 1982.

Carter, Mary Ellen and William McGarey, M.D. *Edgar Cayce on Healing.* New York, New York: Warner Books, Inc., 1969.

Chang, Stephen, M.D. *The Complete System of Self-Healing Internal Exercises*. San Francisco, California: Tao Publishing, 1986.

Compton, Madonna Sophia. *Herbal Gold*. St. Paul, Minnesota: Llewellyn Publications, 2000.

Cummings, Stephen, F.N.P. and Dana Ullman, M.P.H. *Everybody's Guide to Homeopathic Medicines*. Jeremy P. Tarcher, Inc., Los Angeles, 1984

Denning, Melita and Osborne Phillips. *The Llewellyn Practical Guide to Creative Visualization*. St. Paul, Minnesota: Llewellyn Publications, 1983.

Editors of *Prevention Magazine. Understanding Vitamins and Minerals*. Emmaus, Pennsylvania: Rodale Press Inc., 1984.

————*Pain Free*. Emmaus, Pennsylvania: Rodale Press Inc., 1986.

————*Fighting Disease*. Emmaus, Pennsylvania: Rodale Press Inc., 1984.

————*Natural Weight Loss*. Emmaus, Pennsylvania: Rodale Press Inc., 1985.

————*Everyday Health Hints*. Emmaus, Pennsylvania: Rodale Press Inc., 1985.

Fox, Michael W., M.D. *The Healing Touch*. New York, New York: Newmarket Press, 1981.

Bibliography

Frazier, Anitra and Norma Eckroate. *The Natural Cat—A Holistic Guide for Finicky Owners.* New York, New York: Kampmann Publishing Co., 1981.

Griffin, Judy, Ph.D. *Mother Nature's Herbal.* St. Paul, Minnesota: Llewellyn Publications, 1997.

Guyton, Arthur C., M.D. *Textbook of Medical Physiology.* Philadelphia, Pennsylvania: W. B. Saunders Co., 1981.

Hay, Louise L. *You Can Heal Your Life.* Santa Monica, California: Hay House, 1999.

Heinerman, John. *The Complete Book of Spices: Their Medical, Nutritional and Culinary Uses.* New Canaan, Connecticut: Keats Publishing, Inc., 1983.

Herbal Almanac for the Year 2000. St. Paul, Minnesota: Llewellyn Publications, 1999.

Isselbacher et al. *Harrison's Principles of Internal Medicine.* New York, New York: McGraw Hill Book Co., 1980.

Lu, Henry C. *Chinese System of Food. Cures Prevention and Remedies.* New York, New York: Sterling Publishing Co. Inc., 1986.

Mills, Simon, M.A. *The Dictionary of Modern Herbalism.* New York, New York: Thorsons Publishing Group, 1985.

Monahan, Evelyn M. *The Miracle of Metaphysical Healing.* West Nyack, New York: Parker Publishing Co. Inc., 1975.

Nugent, Nancy, ed. *Prevention Magazine. Food and Nutrition.* Emmaus, Pennsylvania: Rodale Press Inc., 1983.

Panos, Maesimund, M.D. and Jane Heimlich. *Homeopathic Medicine at Home.* Los Angeles, California: Jeremy P. Tarcher, Inc., 1980.

Pelletier, Kenneth. *Mind As Healer Mind As Slayer.* New York, New York: Dell Publishing Co., Inc., 1977.

Pitcairn, Richard, D.V.M. and Susan Pitcairn. *Dr. Pitcairn's Complete Guide to Natural Health for Dogs and Cats.* Emmaus, Pennsylvania: Rodale Press, 1982.

Read, Anne, Carol Ilstrup, and Margaret Gammon. *Edgar Cayce on Diet and Health.* New York, New York: Warner Books, Inc., 1969.

Reilly, Harold and Ruth Hagy Brod. *The Edgar Cayce Handbook for Health Through Drugless Therapy.* New York, New York: The Berkley Publishing Group, Inc., 1975.

Roman, Sanaya. *Living With Joy.* Tiburon, California: H. J. Kramer Inc., 1986.

Royal, Penny C. *Herbally Yours.* Provo, Utah: Sound Nutrition, 1982.

The Biochemic Handbook. St. Louis, Missouri: Formur, Inc. Publishers, 1976.

Walker, N. W. *Fresh Vegetable and Fruit Juices.* Prescott, Arizona: Norwalk Press Publishers, 1978.

Weiss, Gaea and Shandor Weiss. *Growing & Using the Healing Herbs.* Rodale Press Inc., Emmaus, Penn., 1985.

Index

Index

Index

senility, 153, 172

sinus, 2–3, 57, 131, 148

sodium, 109, 115, 124–125

solar plexus, 32–33, 159

soybean, 115

spastic colon, 34

sprouts, 119, 126–127

stress, 19, 26, 32, 34, 45, 80–81, 85–95, 110, 158

sugar, 66, 101, 103–105, 111, 118, 121, 132

T

telepathy, 50

thymus gland, 21–22, 56, 82, 187

tofu, 115–116, 124

toxins, 48, 87, 117, 122, 128–129, 145, 158

trace elements, 125

U

ulcers, 45, 85, 129, 133, 148–149, 159

V

vaginal infection, 10, 129

visualization, 3, 35, 45–47, 50–53, 55, 57–59, 61, 141, 154, 187, 189

vitamins, 101, 103, 106, 111–112, 115, 119, 122–123, 126–127, 135, 148, 154, 167, 181

vitamin A, 126, 134

vitamin C, 109, 123–124, 127, 178

vitamin D, 110, 124, 127

vitamin E, 111, 127

vitamin K, 127

vitamin B, 112, 127

W

weight, xiii, xiv, 32–33, 98–99, 139, 183

white light, 3, 16, 26, 32–33, 55–56, 59, 81, 159, 181, 183, 187

Y

yogurt, 108, 116, 126–127

Z

zinc, 115, 119, 125, 167

REACH FOR THE MOON

Llewellyn publishes hundreds of books on your favorite subjects! To get these exciting books, including the ones on the following pages, check your local bookstore or order them directly from Llewellyn.

ORDER BY PHONE

- Call toll-free within the U.S. and Canada, 1-800-THE MOON
- In Minnesota, call (651) 291-1970
- We accept VISA, MasterCard, and American Express

ORDER BY MAIL

- Send the full price of your order (MN residents add 7% sales tax) in U.S. funds, plus postage & handling to:

  Llewellyn Worldwide
  P.O. Box 64383, Dept. (K 427-8)
  St. Paul, MN 55164–0383, U.S.A.

POSTAGE & HANDLING

(For the U.S., Canada, and Mexico)

- $4.00 for orders $15.00 and under
- $5.00 for orders over $15.00
- No charge for orders over $100.00

We ship UPS in the continental United States. We ship standard mail to P.O. boxes. Orders shipped to Alaska, Hawaii, The Virgin Islands, and Puerto Rico are sent first-class mail. Orders shipped to Canada and Mexico are sent surface mail.

International orders: Airmail—add freight equal to price of each book to the total price of order, plus $5.00 for each non-book item (audio tapes, etc.).

Surface mail—Add $1.00 per item.

Allow 2 weeks for delivery on all orders.
Postage and handling rates subject to change.

DISCOUNTS

We offer a 20% discount to group leaders or agents. You must order a minimum of 5 copies of the same book to get our special quantity price.

FREE CATALOG

Get a free copy of our color catalog, New Worlds of Mind and Spirit. Subscribe for just $10.00 in the United States and Canada ($30.00 overseas, airmail). Many bookstores carry New Worlds—ask for it!

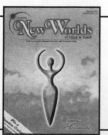

Visit our website at www.llewellyn.com for more information.

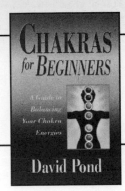

Chakras for Beginners
A Guide to Balancing Your Chakra Energies

DAVID POND

The chakras are spinning vortexes of energy located just in front of your spine and positioned from the tailbone to the crown of the head. They are a map of your inner world—your relationship to yourself and how you experience energy. They are also the batteries for the various levels of your life energy. The freedom with which energy can flow back and forth between you and the universe correlates directly to your total health and well-being.

Blocks to this energy flow can manifest itself as disease, discomfort, lack of energy, fear, or an emotional imbalance. By acquainting yourself with the chakra system, learning how they work and how they should operate optimally, you can perceive your own blocks and restrictions and develop guidelines for relieving entanglements.

The chakras stand out as the most useful model for you to identify how your energy is expressing itself. With *Chakras for Beginners* you will discover what is causing any imbalances, how to bring your energies back into alignment, and how to achieve higher levels of consciousness.

1-56718-537-1
216 pp., 5³⁄₁₆ x 8   **$9.95**

To order, call 1-800-THE MOON
Prices subject to change without notice

Numerology for Beginners
Easy Guide to Love • Money • Destiny

GERIE BAUER

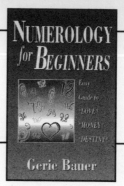

Every letter and number in civilization has a particular power, or vibration. For centuries, people have read these vibrations through the practice of numerology. References in the Bible even describe Jesus using numerology to change the names of his disciples. *Numerology for Beginners* is a quick ready-to-use reference that lets you find your personal vibrations based on the numbers associated with your birthdate and name.

Within minutes, you will be able to assess the vibrations surrounding a specific year, month, and day—even a specific person. Detect whether you're in a business cycle or a social cycle, and whether a certain someone or occupation would be compatible with you. Plus, learn to detect someone's personality within seconds of learning their first name!

1-56718-057-4
336 pp., 5³⁄₁₆ x 8, softcover $9.95